★
NORTH
STAR
WAY

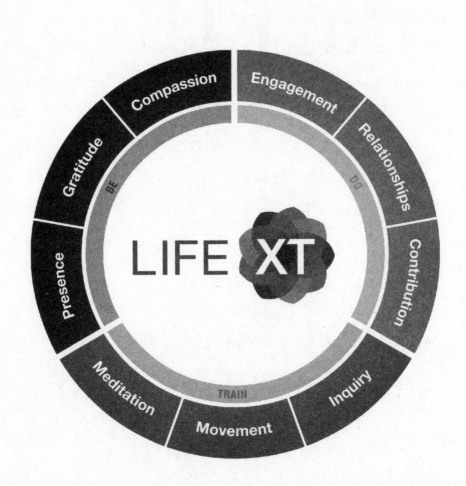

Start Here

Master the Lifelong Habit
of Wellbeing

Eric Langshur
and Nate Klemp, PhD

Foreword by Dr. Richard J. Davidson

NORTH STAR WAY

New York   London   Toronto   Sydney   New Delhi

North Star Way
An Imprint of Simon & Schuster, Inc.
1230 Avenue of the Americas
New York, NY 10020

First North Star Way hardcover edition May 2016

NORTH STAR WAY and colophon are trademarks of Simon & Schuster, Inc.

For information about special discounts for bulk purchases, please contact
Simon & Schuster Special Sales at 1-866-506-1949 or business@simonandschuster.com.

The North Star Way Speakers Bureau can bring authors to your live event.
For more information or to book an event, contact the North Star Way Speakers Bureau
at 1-212-698-8888 or visit our website at www.thenorthstarway.com.

Manufactured in the United States of America

10 9 8 7 6 5 4 3 2 1

Library of Congress Cataloging-in-Publication Data

Names: Langshur, Eric, author. | Klemp, Nathaniel J., 1979 author.
Title: Start here : master the lifelong habit of wellbeing / by Eric
    Langshur and Nate Klemp.
Description: New York : North Star Way, 2016. | Includes bibliographical
    references and index.
Identifiers: LCCN 2015043325 (print) | LCCN 2015047762 (ebook) | ISBN
    9781501129087 (hardback) | ISBN 9781501129148 ()
Subjects: LCSH: Happiness. | Stress management. | Mental health. |
    Satisfaction. | Wellbeing. | BISAC: SELF-HELP / Personal Growth /
    Happiness. | HEALTH & FITNESS / Healthy Living. | SELF-HELP / Stress
    Management.
Classification: LCC BF575.H27 L364 2016 (print) | LCC BF575.H27 (ebook) | DDC
    158—dc23
LC record available at http://lccn.loc.gov/2015043325

ISBN 978-1-5011-2908-7
ISBN 978-1-5011-2914-8 (ebook)

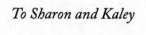

To Sharon and Kaley

Contents

Foreword

BY DR. RICHARD J. DAVIDSON

Today, an increasingly large percentage of the population has begun to notice the lack of emotional balance in their lives: They are stressed at work and find themselves moody and volatile. They feel less than optimal physically. They spend less time than they would like with their families, yet when they are with their spouse or children, the interaction is often marred by interpersonal discord. These same people are searching for strategies to help them become less stressed and calmer. If you are one of those people, *Start Here* will help you find the set of tools you need to begin making meaningful changes in your life.

The genius of *Start Here* is that it is not just a book. It presents a training program called Life Cross Training (LIFE XT) that contains specific exercises for your mind and body designed to help you improve your life and enable your sense of wellbeing to flourish. *Start Here* provides a wealth of helpful information grounded in contemporary scientific research. It offers additional resources for those wishing to probe specific areas more deeply and, most important, a program of concrete exercises you can use to help transform your everyday life and create a stronger and more enduring sense of happiness.

One of the many things I like about the approach of the LIFE XT program is that it is not limited to the ancient contemplative practices, such as meditation. While I myself have benefited enormously from such practices, it is clear that the other two pillars of happiness training contained within the LIFE XT approach are critically needed: movement and inquiry. Movement includes both aerobic and nonaerobic forms of exercise. The scientific evidence concerning the benefits of physical exercise, particularly for the brain, is now very robust and compelling, and the practical advice and recommendations in *Start Here* will be enormously helpful to those who have not yet incorporated regular physical activity into their routine.

The Inquiry piece of the LIFE XT training provides an important tool for questioning the validity and veracity of stressful thoughts. This practice has the power to unravel the many stressful stories that keep us from experiencing happiness: *I have too much to do. My husband isn't there for me. I don't have enough.*

The three foundational practices of LIFE XT (Meditation, Movement, and Inquiry) are intended to become part of a weekly routine; they require setting aside time and attention. The second part of the LIFE XT program consists of six Be and Do Stage practices. Unlike the first three practices, these practices are designed to cultivate qualities like presence, gratitude, compassion, engagement, relationships, and contribution. The recommendations contained in this section again derive from many different sources: some from the ancient wisdom traditions, some from positive psychology, and others from more rigorous neuroscientific research. As someone who knows this space both as a scientist and as a practitioner, I found the assembly of this wide range of material in a single location—presented in a highly readable and practical format—to be very helpful.

The book's foundation rests not only on ancient wisdom traditions but also on modern science. Important studies such as the recent findings on "mind wandering" by Matthew Killingsworth and Daniel Gilbert at Harvard University provide a useful framework for the average person to understand how these practices actually serve to rewire the brain in ways that decrease stress and increase overall wellbeing. This kind of information can be very helpful and inspiring as people begin to make positive changes in their lives.

The sources of insight that guide the recommendations set forth in *Start Here* do not emanate from a single tradition, a particular method, or a specific theoretical orientation. Instead, it is a comprehensive framework that combines the best practices from many different wisdom traditions, from modern science, and from philosophy, and applies them in a very practical program for improving everyday life. The result is an integrated set of tools that can be deployed in a simple way to enhance wellbeing.

For these reasons, I believe this book and the program that is presented will benefit anyone seeking to live with greater happiness. I urge you to investigate the application of the many simple practices that are offered up in this book to your daily life, and to stick with them and continue to implement them. It is only through regular practice that the brain will change, and modern science now clearly indicates that this can indeed happen.

May you find this book helpful and may you improve your life by adopting these practices.

—Dr. Richard J. Davidson, William James and Vilas Professor of Psychology and Psychiatry at the University of Wisconsin; director of the Waisman Lab for Brain Imaging and Behavior and the Lab for Affective Neuroscience; founder and chair of the Center for Investigating Healthy Minds

THE OPEN SECRET

An Introduction to Life Cross Training

There's a truth we've learned to embrace—one that has changed our lives and led us to bring the idea of training wellbeing to thousands of people. We call this truth the Open Secret.

You likely already know this "secret." Think about people you admire, those who seem like they have everything life has to offer: a beautiful home, a great family, and ongoing opportunities. From what you can see, they have it all.

Here's the secret: Scratch the surface of what looks like success, and chances are you will find a person who has experienced a mixture of highs and lows, moments of deep contentment along with moments of sadness, anger, anxiety, and fear. The fact is that while most of us project a polished facade, we all search for happiness, fulfillment, and joy as we work to navigate the challenges and obstacles that life brings us.

This is likely true of the people you admire. It's probably true of you. It is certainly true of us.

I am Eric Langshur.

For most of my adult life, I started each day with the same harrowing morning ritual: Wake up. Eyes open. Brain on. Then immediately, the assault of thoughts would begin:

What have I got to get done today? What balls am I in danger of dropping? What is Elizabeth thinking about what I said to her yesterday? I need to remember to call my dad. I should hurry or I'm going to be late for work.

On and on . . . and on.

The experience was so normal to me that I wasn't even aware it was happening. Somewhere around my fortieth birthday, though, I did start to notice this unrelenting stream of thoughts, and I realized, *This voice in my head is exhausting me.*

Clearly, this wasn't the kind of joy-filled life I once thought I would be living when I achieved "success," and this realization of my incessant inner dialogue wasn't anything like the kind of "waking up" epiphany that the mystics describe. Instead, becoming acutely aware of my thoughts, worries, and anxieties only intensified the ever-present undercurrent of stress in my life. As a corporate executive and serial entrepreneur, I knew how to build businesses and manage large organizations. But, I began to realize, I didn't know how to manage my own mind.

This jarring insight set me on a decade-long search to understand how to be happier. I sought wisdom by reading the great spiritual texts: the Old and New Testaments, the Quran, the Bhagavad Gita, and the texts of Taoism and Buddhism. These in turn sparked an interest in philosophy, turning me toward the Greeks (Plato, Aristotle, Epictetus), the Romans (Marcus Aurelius, Seneca), the modern Europeans (Nietzsche, Goethe, Kierkegaard), and the American Transcendentalists (Thoreau, Emerson).

I became a philosophy and self-help junkie in my search for meaning. My wife, Sharon, regularly laughed at my enthusiastic exploration of this literature. My head reeled with the plethora of ancient wisdom and advice on wellbeing, and I experimented, bouncing from idea to idea during an amazing period of transformation.

Very slowly, two incredible developments emerged. My mind started to quiet, and after years of deep exploration and study, I began to see that these great spiritual and philosophical tomes shared a similar set of ideas about happiness and wellbeing.

I am Nate Klemp.

At age twenty-seven, I had my life turned upside down.

In the final year of my PhD program at Princeton, one warm September afternoon, my wife and I were riding our bikes side by side, lost in conversation. We didn't notice as we veered toward each other—until our handlebars locked together at full speed.

CRACK. I heard the spokes in my front wheel shatter as my handlebars twisted uncontrollably. I launched forward headfirst onto the gravel path.

Five seconds later I lay on the ground, staring up at the blue sky, my head, neck, and jaw throbbing, my wife leaning over me.

One month later I began to feel the full effects of the injuries to my head, neck, and jaw. The Princeton campus began to feel like a ship traversing rough seas. My world started spinning. My ears rang. Something wasn't right.

Four months later my mental and physical condition had gone from bad to worse. Before the accident, I was a happily married, fit, razor-sharp graduate student at Princeton. Now the physical and mental aftershocks of my accident left me struggling to perform even the most mundane tasks. Picking up groceries felt exhausting. Two hours of writing my dissertation felt like twelve. A three-hour flight felt like a trip around the world. My entire life felt like I was running a marathon at mile 25. But there was no finish line in sight.

Until then the biggest challenges I had faced were theoretical. As a grad student in political philosophy, I spent long days at the library, working to understand political rhetoric, inequality, and other abstract questions. Now my challenges were practical and deeply personal. *How can I part these clouds of anxiety and fatigue? How can I save my marriage? How can I salvage my career? How can I train my body and mind to live a better life?*

Answering these questions became my passion in life. I used my training in philosophy to search the texts throughout the ages for answers. These readings led me to a new set of life practices. I learned to meditate. I became an avid practitioner of yoga. Soon, my career ambitions shifted outside the conventional academic path, from tenure to wellbeing, from the theory of happiness to its practice. After years spent understanding philosophy as a set of ideas, I now wanted to experience philosophy as a way of life.

Life Cross Training

So began the work of Life Cross Training (LIFE XT). Like many people on the journey of self-discovery, we each felt lost in a sea of conflicting insights, ideas, and programs. Then fortuitously we met and discovered each of us had separately followed a similar path, studying many of the same texts, coming to similar conclusions.

Sorting through this maze of wisdom and advice on how to live a better life became our deep passion. Our hunger for greater wellbeing worked like rocket fuel to motivate us to bring together the most powerful ideas and practices for achieving wellbeing and happiness.

We began with ancient wisdom. For thousands of years, after all, philosophers and spiritual teachers have put forth wisdom and ideas for living a better life. To guide our journeys, we decided to create a map—a framework that would synthesize this expansive body of ancient wisdom. With the help of leading experts in classics, philosophy, and religious studies, we explored the vast array of practical advice offered by the great philosophical traditions of the East and West. While we found differences in doctrine and practice, we also found a powerful underlying set of shared insights. Just about every tradition converged on certain core practices: presence, gratitude, compassion, contribution, and more. You will find the most potent of these in the nine practices of LIFE XT.

Then we started to live these practices, comparing our experiences as we journeyed on. We turned the gym in Eric's home into a training room for happiness and wellbeing, writing out the early LIFE XT framework on the walls, reviewing our results, and weaving the pertinent practices into our daily lives.

As we developed our daily practice, we looked to advances in the fields of neuroscience and positive psychology, where we found scientific validation for the synthesized framework we had developed. Working closely with Dr. John Cacioppo, the pioneer of the field of social neuroscience, Dr. Richard Davidson, the preeminent researcher on the neuroscience of meditation, and other leading scientists highlighted throughout this book, we researched the vast body of evidence to support the LIFE XT practices. We were excited to discover that the benefits of these timeless practices were grounded in hard scientific fact.

These ancient insights and modern scientific discoveries captivated and inspired us. They helped us develop a more optimistic picture of what it is to be human and how all of us can live a good life. True, we all face constant challenges but, we discovered, with the right practices and applied effort, anyone can learn how to train this essential life skill of wellbeing.

Nate recalls how his body and mind changed as a result of this training:

My posture shifted from slumped to upright. I had more energy and felt more at ease. My mind also changed. This new training in happiness didn't eliminate negative emotions like sadness, fear, and shame, but it created a subtle sense of space around them. It helped me learn how to stay in the fire of even the most uncomfortable states without having them overtake my life. These benefits rippled through all areas of my life. I felt a deeper sense of purpose in my career, more connected to my friends and family, and more present in my marriage. Through it all, my life became richer, more meaningful, and above all, happier.

Eric had a similar experience:

Although I continued to hear the unremitting voice in my head, it no longer gripped me in its manic swirl the way it it once did. Over time, a peaceful spaciousness developed inside me and I began to witness my thoughts—watching them come and go without getting caught in their often painful hold. I was thrilled to realize that I was actually developing the skill of attention, actively choosing where to place my focus. This simple skill has given rise to profound changes in my life, making me more joyful, more productive, and a better husband, parent, son, colleague, and friend.

Now, years later, LIFE XT has been adopted by thousands of people seeking to optimize their lives as well as companies dedicated to elevating their employees to peak performance, including top law firms, digital media agencies, and venture capital firms. Through our individual, group, and corporate training programs, we have helped people enhance their wellbeing, with dramatic and lasting results. *Start Here*—the book you are holding—will lead you to these same discoveries.

Life's Challenges

Start Here begins with the Open Secret: the simple truth that we all encounter a myriad of challenges and obstacles as we move throughout our lives. In everyday life, we easily lose sight of the fact that everyone struggles. Turn on the TV and we see attractive celebrities who seem to have it all together and commercials that spark fantasies about how good life would be with a new car, bigger house, or more attractive mate. Log on to Facebook or Twitter and we mostly see a similarly idealized world—a world full of vacation photos, professional triumphs, and peak moments such as getting engaged, having a child, or getting married.

In this selectively sunny world, other people don't get stressed, feel anxious, or spend their days running worst-case scenarios in their minds. But of course *no one* actually lives in that world. Picture-perfect celebrities struggle and experience the very same negative emotions that the rest of us do. That friend who just returned from Maui is already back in her daily rut of stress and irritation. The handsome, blissful couple with all the glossy wedding photographs went through months of anxiety planning the event, and may spend years stressing over how to pay it off. While we may not talk about it openly, the truth is that everyone experiences difficult moments.

Take Andrea, for example, a dedicated LIFE XT practitioner. On the outside, she looks as though she has it all: She's a successful entrepreneur, a high-powered corporate executive, and a respected community leader. But she, like everyone else, has a powerful narrative about the challenges she has faced in life:

> *Growing up, life was uncomplicated and somewhat predictable. My summers were spent waitressing at the Jersey Shore, waiting for Bruce Springsteen to show up while my friends hung out. I felt safe and loved. I earned my degree in social work and set out to change the world! At thirty-one, I fell in love and got married. But less than two years later, life started to throw me curveballs. My parents died within six months of each other, the doctors told us that our second daughter might never walk, and our finances became a concern as medical bills mounted. Joy and optimism shifted to anxiety, depression, and a fear of what's next. I was working 24/7, blaming others for my unhappiness, and seeing no light at the end of the tunnel—I shut down and became numb. It was years later, when I experienced a bad case of vertigo, that I was forced to begin to untangle the web.*

Like Andrea, we all have a story and a deep desire to improve our lives. Of course this insight isn't new. The nature of human dissatisfaction and the quest for greater happiness is part of the human condition. Now, though, our modern age presents us with a unique set of challenges that can make wellbeing seem especially elusive.

Consider just a few of the most pressing challenges in our modern lives. Stress has become a way of life for many of us. According to the American Psychological Association, 70 percent of Americans report that they experience physical or nonphysical symptoms of stress, and 80 percent say their stress level has increased or stayed the same over the last year.[1] Stress also makes us sick: The American Institute of Stress estimates that more than half of all visits to primary care physicians are for stress-related complaints.[2]

While smartphones, tablets, and other technologies have improved our lives in countless ways, these tools also pose a deep challenge to our wellbeing. They consume our time and attention. The average adult spends more than eleven hours a day exposed to electronic media (TV, radio, computer, etc.), and checks his or her phone more than 150 times a day, which makes it difficult to focus, work, and be present with the people we care about.[3]

Add to this the speed of our modern lives. We now move through the day at a dizzying pace. We can communicate more in an hour than our grandparents could in a week. We can, for example, stand in line for coffee while attending an important meeting via conference call, emailing our friends, and catching up on the latest headlines. This warp-speed pace makes it difficult to slow down and simply be present in the moments of our lives.

It's not just the stress, technology, and speed of the external world that challenges our wellbeing. It's also our human biology that shapes the way we react to these external conditions. Our brains, after all, didn't evolve to live in the midst of constant digital distraction—to multitask, write emails, or face the continual low-grade stressors of the modern world. The human brain evolved to handle a much more primitive state of affairs: gathering food, building shelter, and running from the occasional saber-toothed tiger.

This is the real paradox of our modern age: Our bodies and minds simply weren't designed to handle the near-constant stress of the modern world. As we will see in the next chapter, this biological contradiction keeps us in a state of vigilance and anxiety, skewing our thoughts toward the negative and causing our minds to wander for about 50 percent of our waking hours.[4] In short, we are biologically wired to experience the very opposite of happiness and wellbeing.

Hope for Happiness

Fundamentally, we are all seeking to be happier. The problem is that there are so many different books, programs, and systems for living a better life that it's easy to become overwhelmed by the vast array of conflicting approaches. This was our experience. In the development of LIFE XT, we explored bestselling books on happiness that made big promises. But we found that within a few weeks, or even a few days, after turning the final page, we returned to our old habits and began searching for the next book, system, or seminar. While we uncovered many amazing tools and insights, we didn't find any comprehensive programs that offered a clear road map to wellbeing. We also simply didn't know what to believe. Many of these books and programs were based on intuition and personal experience—not scientific evidence.

In the end, we found that most programs presented wellbeing as something that *happens* in an instant—a kind of "get-happy-quick" approach. But we knew from our own lives and from the vast body of emerging research in neuroscience that happiness doesn't spring from an idea or a flash of insight; wellbeing is a *skill* that must be trained, and this training has the power to change the brain.[5]

This idea may sound obvious, but it is truly revolutionary. Until just recently, most scientists viewed altering the structure of the brain through training our ability to direct our attention as impossible. The adult brain was considered to be fixed, resistant to change. Recent discoveries have led researchers to revise this understanding of a fixed brain, and we now know that the adult brain is capable of change throughout our lives. Just as we exercise to train our bodies and increase physical fitness, we can train our brains to optimize wellbeing.

A New Kind of Program

Inspired by this emerging science of neuroplasticity, the insights of ancient wisdom, and the encouragement of countless friends and colleagues, we set out to create a different kind of program—a comprehensive training system for wellbeing grounded in rigorous research. LIFE XT is based on three core insights, drawn from this research:

- *Training.* Wellbeing is a skill that can be trained.
- *Attention.* We can develop this skill by learning to direct our attention, which shapes our experience of life.
- *Integration.* The ordinary moments of everyday life offer the ultimate training ground for this practice of wellbeing.

LIFE XT is a comprehensive training program for complete wellbeing designed around these themes. The program consists of three stages with three practices each. You will develop one practice at a time, and at the end of each stage, you will measure your progress using the LIFE XT assessment tool. Nine practices may sound like a lot, but we have designed LIFE XT for maximum efficiency so that you can minimize the amount of time you need to devote to these practices by integrating them into your everyday life.

To help you cultivate this new way of life, *Start Here* offers step-by-step instructions. Think of it like P90X[6] for the soul—a structured program designed to help you develop physical, mental, and emotional fitness. The program also provides access to a cutting-edge assessment tool designed in close collaboration with Drs. John and Stephanie Cacioppo at the University of Chicago to help you track your practice and measure your progress. This human analytics platform will allow you to see how these practices have an impact on just about every aspect of your life: happiness, energy level, focus, stress, sleep, health, and more.

As the LIFE XT program becomes integrated into your daily life, you will find yourself more at ease, waking up each day to the moment-to-moment feeling of being fulfilled, fully engaged in the world that surrounds you, quietly content with your life and conscious of its blessing. In short, you will be happier.

Welcome to LIFE XT. Your journey starts here.

The Biological Challenge of Being Human

As a species, we didn't evolve to communicate electronically over great distances, search through cyberspace for information, live in vertical housing, or commute in individual vehicles. In the beginning, we were hunters and gatherers, and yes, we were also prey.

Imagine you are traversing the African savanna in search of your next meal. It's very hot; there's been no rain for months. As you walk through the tall grass, you hear a snapping sound—something is lurking behind you. You freeze. Your eyes dart around but you see nothing.

Out of nowhere, a lioness springs toward you, jaws open and claws sharp. You run as fast as you can, zigzagging through the grass, barely managing to escape. For the next hour, you live in fear. Your heart is pounding; your mind is racing with worry about how you're going to get back to your family alive, and whether the lion is still out there or is heading for your village. . . .

This may sound like a scene from a National Geographic documentary, but Stanford University neurobiologist Robert Sapolsky argues that such scenarios give us a profound insight into the problems we twenty-first-century humans face in everyday life.[1] Although our lives bear little resemblance to those of our ancient ancestors, our brains and bodies remain wired to deal with precisely these kinds of prehistoric situations.

Today's challenge is that our modern lifestyle has evolved in the opposite direction. Day after day, we face stressors that are not life-threatening but "psychological and social"[2]—arising from work, relationships, and a constant deluge of information and digital distraction our prehistoric ancestors could scarcely have imagined.

Prehistoric Instincts—Modern Worries

The lion in the savanna scenario illustrates the paradox of being human in the modern era: *We are running complex software on prehistoric hardware.* The machinery of our mind and body was built for running from lions. It was designed to handle intense momentary stress followed by longer periods of rest and recovery. It was not designed to handle the constant low-grade stress we navigate every day.

Today it's not our physical survival we worry about but our *social* survival: impressing our colleagues at work, paying down mortgages, or staying attractive for our partner. Our struggle for social survival produces a cascade of thinking that starts the instant we wake up and only quiets in exquisite moments—during moments of intense love, time spent in nature, or experiences of prayer and meditation. Otherwise this stream of thought runs continuously throughout the day, ceasing only when we drift into sleep.

Here's how one LIFE XT participant, Heidi, an account manager at a digital media agency, describes her experience of this endless stream of thinking:

I'm the daughter of an overly skeptical, trust-no-one father and an anxiety-ridden, overachieving mother. Even though I think they're the best parents in the world, it's no wonder I spend every day and night worrying about every little thing. The older I get, the heavier my decisions weigh, and I've found myself paralyzed with doubt and worry more often than not. Did I do enough? Was it good enough? Did I move too fast? Did I wait too long? What does everybody else think? *Constant doubt invades my thinking. It never stops. I can (and will) get myself worked up over anything.*

Heidi is not alone in experiencing doubt and anxiety. The specific worries that people describe may be different, but the experience is universal. And it's one that cuts to the core of this modern paradox: We react to finances, workplace drama, relationship conflict, and the many other social stressors of modern life as if our very survival were under threat. In response to our stressful thoughts, our bodies and minds activate the same primitive response mechanisms. Our breath shortens, our muscles tighten, and stress hormones like adrenaline, norepinephrine, and cortisol flood the body. We prepare to fight, freeze, or flee, as though we just encountered a grizzly bear on a remote mountain trail. And unlike our ancestors who had time to rest and recover, many of us spend almost every waking hour living with the burden of never-ending stress.

Wired for the Negative

Our body's response to stress is just the beginning of the challenges we face. Our minds have also evolved with a *negativity bias*—a tendency to live in a state of vigilance and anxiety, running negative simulations of past regret or future harm and remembering the bad instead of the good.[3] Neuropsychologist Rick Hanson outlines several ways in which our neurobiology shapes our experience (for more on these biological forces, see Appendix 2: The Triune Brain).

- *Vigilance and anxiety.* In its default state, our brain remains attentive to potential threats, constantly gathering information from both sensory inputs and memories. This biologically driven instinct can turn coworkers into rivals and the driver who just cut you off in traffic into a dangerous enemy. Being vigilant and alert kept our ancestors hyperaware of their surroundings and ready for a surprise attack. But in the relative safety of the modern world, this evolved instinct can create counterproductive thoughts and behaviors.

- *High-priority storage.* "Your brain is like Velcro for the negative experiences and Teflon for the positive ones," writes Hanson.[4] Have you ever noticed how peak moments such as great dinners, romantic walks, and profound insights are easily forgotten, whereas intense anxiety, grief, and emotional traumas stay with us for years? In evolutionary terms, this focus on the negative makes sense. It's much more important for long-term survival to remember that a deadly snake lives behind that rock than to remember the lovely flowers it lives amongst. Yet in our current world, this bias toward the negative leaves us largely thinking about the things that went wrong, and makes us less likely to pay attention to the sunrise, the joy in a child's laughter, or the feeling of gratitude for the many good things in our lives.

- *Negative simulations of the future.* In addition to impacting memories, our brain's negativity bias shapes our projections of the future.[5] Our brain is constantly running simulations about what might happen to help us anticipate future dangers that might threaten our survival. It's what keeps us awake at three a.m., churning through future worst-case scenarios. In prehistoric times, it might have been helpful to think through how best to escape from predators, but in modern life this biologically driven tendency can leave us worrying about a disagreement with a coworker or imagining increasingly far-fetched, worst-case scenarios about life's challenges (money, job, spouse, status, or reputation).

We're All Wired This Way . . .

These neurobiologically driven instincts make our lives quite challenging. They can turn anticipating a ten-minute speech we have to give into what feels like a near-death experience. They can turn a disagreement with our partner into all-consuming drama. Simply put, our default biological wiring creates obstacles to our well-being.

And yet the widespread denial of this basic biological fact makes matters even worse. Most of us, after all, spend our days hiding the effects of these powerful instincts—more or less out of necessity. Few people show up in a social setting and say, "I've been so stressed at work lately that I'm having panic attacks." Almost nobody walks into their boss's office and says, "I come to work each day feeling like my life has no real meaning." Instead, most of us live in a world where such feelings are carefully tucked away out of sight.

Your Biologically Driven Set Point

This biological wiring that works in the shadows of the modern world establishes what scientists call the *happiness set point*. The set point is the unique spot that each of us occupies on the spectrum of life satisfaction: high, low, or somewhere in between. Think of it as your default location on the spectrum of wellbeing. On good days, you may rise above your set point. On bad days, you may fall below it. But research shows that, in the absence of sustained conscious effort, you will almost always return to the default location of your happiness set point.

Lottery winners, for example, experience a momentary increase in happiness after winning, but within a few months their happiness levels return to their original set point (psychologists call this phenomenon *hedonic adaptation*). Accident victims experience a dramatic drop in happiness after tragedy strikes, but over the long run they report returning to happiness levels only slightly lower than their original set point.[6] Whether you experience a devastating loss or win a million dollars, after about a year, your ratio of good moods to bad will likely return to about the same level as before: your original set point.

The power of these forces holds huge implications for our understanding of wellbeing. It means that much of what we hear about happiness is simply not true. We have all encountered books, programs, or infomercials that promise quick fixes for a happier life. We have all heard songs like "Don't Worry, Be Happy" or the "Happy" song, and while they may momentarily give us a lift in mood, they rarely influence our happiness set point. Science tells us it's just not that easy. It's nearly impossible to just wake up one day and decide to be happy.

The good news is that it is possible to reset our set point. But it requires training. This training begins by understanding the three forces that determine the location of the set point: judgment, attachment, and resistance.

Understanding the Set Point Forces

Imagine that you're late for an important commitment. You jump in the car and pull out in a rush. As you turn onto the road, you find yourself behind a slow-moving car. Now the three impulses of the mind—the set point forces—spring into action. You immediately *judge* the other person to be a horrible driver. You *attach* to your own reputation as a punctual person. You *resist* the situation by feeling stressed. In this moment, as in almost every moment, these three set point forces shape your thoughts and experiences.

The Three Set Point Forces

1. *Judgment* is the mind's tendency to divide the inner and outer world into categories—good/bad, right/wrong, like/dislike.
2. *Attachment* is the mind's tendency to approach or cling to pleasurable thoughts, beliefs, or sensations.
3. *Resistance* is the mind's tendency to fight or flee from painful sensations, experiences, or situations.

Judgment: The First Set Point Force

Judgment helps us make sense of the world by sorting our experiences into the conceptual boxes of good/bad, right/wrong, like/dislike. For our survival, judgment is a necessary capacity: money = like, disease = bad, stealing = wrong. So it's natural that, as thoughts, sensations, and emotions arise, the mind instantly begins to judge. When we look in the mirror, talk to a friend, go to a restaurant, or read the newspaper, our minds churn out constant judgments. We might look "good," our friend might be "lost," the food might be "terrible," and the news "unsettling." We use many words to describe our judgments, but they all boil down to the simple dichotomy of good and bad.

While necessary for survival, judgment sits at the root of much of our inner turmoil. In the *Tao Te Ching* as translated by Stephen Mitchell, a text that dates back to the sixth century BCE, Lao-tzu observed:

> *When people see some things as beautiful,*
> *other things become ugly.*
> *When people see some things as good,*
> *other things become bad.*[7]

Judgment, in other words, divides our world, leading us to attach to the "good" and resist the "bad." This biological instinct serves an important purpose: It simplifies the complexity of life, and it helps us hold on to the things that seem beneficial and avoid the things that seem to pose the greatest threat to our survival. But it also limits our experience and creates dissatisfaction. When everything falls on one side or the other, our perspective narrows. We see problems instead of possibilities, potential enemies instead of friends.

Consider a seemingly harmless judgment statement such as "the house is messy." This judgment can be quite useful. It can inspire you to do the dishes, sweep the floor, and tidy up. But it can also become a constant source of stress and anxiety. As you become more and more fixated on cleaning up the "mess," crumbs on the floor can trigger a cascade of stress hormones. Your child's dirty dish can incite anger. Soon all you see is the "mess"—you lose sight of the beauty of your home and the gratitude you feel for having a house in the first place.

The judgments that cause us stress vary from person to person, and indeed, from moment to moment, but the impulse to judge is universal. And the results are the same. The things that we judge to be "bad"—gaining weight, losing money, losing our health—trigger our prehistoric impulses. In the body and the brain, these "bad" things turn into psychological predators, activating the body's stress response, leaving us worried and on guard, rarely if ever at ease.

Modern science confirms that this tendency of the mind is hardwired into the very functioning of the brain's left hemisphere. Jill Bolte Taylor, a Harvard-trained neuroanatomist and author of *My Stroke of Insight*, explains that our left hemisphere "categorizes information into hierarchies including things that attract us (our likes) or repel us (our dislikes) . . . It keeps us abreast of where we stand on the financial scale, academic scale, honesty scale, generosity-of-spirit scale, and every other scale you can imagine."[8]

Although exquisitely practical, this mechanism, left unchecked, can lead to unhappiness. When combined with the negativity bias of the brain, these endless judgments of "good" and "bad" can leave us focusing on all that is wrong with the world, the people in our lives, and ourselves.

Attachment: The Second Set Point Force

In the second of his Four Noble Truths, the Buddha identifies attachment as the root of all human suffering. "From attachment springs grief," the Buddha declares, "from attachment springs fear; for him who is wholly free from attachment there is no grief, much less fear."[9]

The Buddha's wisdom is profound, and yet attachment serves

the human species in many ways. It keeps parents from abandoning their children, motivates performance on the job, and instills healthy behaviors such as exercising and eating well. But when we allow this biologically driven force of the mind to dominate our thoughts, it can sow the seeds of worry, anger, or sadness and have an unfavorable impact on our wellbeing.

When we judge something to be "good," attachments naturally arise. We become attached to relationships, good health, thoughts, beliefs, and outcomes. We can even become attached to those things that society judges to be "bad"—smoking, abusing drugs, overeating—because they give us pleasure, at least at first.

Like judgment, attachment corresponds to a unique pattern of activation of the left prefrontal region of the brain.[10] While often beneficial, as in the attachment of parents to children, attachment can also create intense suffering and emotional unrest. The problem is that lurking behind every attachment is a desire for some sort of permanence—for the feeling that what we have now or hope to have in the future could last forever. An attractive person might attach to the idea of a lifetime of good looks. An intelligent person might attach to the idea of continued razor-sharp cognition. A rich person might attach to the idea of lifelong wealth.

This is the root of the problem. We're attached to permanence—to clinging to the things we hold most dear—but we live in a world of constant change. Despite our best efforts, everything we cling to will one day slip away. Good looks, intelligence, money, and even life itself is impermanent, constantly changing in ways that we simply cannot control. As a result, at a very basic level, we struggle, continually frustrated by our failure to find permanence in a chaotic, uncontrollable, and impermanent world.

Consider love and approval. Many of us cling to the relationships we have or to our ideas about the relationships we should have. Our attachment can create feelings of envy, possessiveness, and resentment. It can leave us fearful that our loved ones might abandon us or terrified that we may never find that special someone we long to have in our lives.

Look closely at your own life and you will likely find this habit of the mind everywhere—in your thoughts about health, death, children, friends, reputation, career, looks—anywhere you believe you have something to lose.

Resistance: The Third Set Point Force

In his third law of motion, the physicist and mathematician Sir Isaac Newton taught that forces always come in pairs. "For every action," he famously declared, "there is an equal and opposite reaction." Newton's law applies in more than the physical realm. It also helps us understand the forces of the set point.

Attachment is a positive force. It draws us toward the things we want to preserve or that we desire. Resistance is the opposite of attachment. When we resist, we pull away: We fight or flee from those experiences we judge to be "bad" in the inner and outer world. Each of us has a unique list of thoughts, sensations, and emotions that cause us to recoil. It might be physical pain, discomfort, the thought of dying, the sight of blood, small spaces, or an encounter with a spider in the bathroom.

The tendency within each of us to resist is normal. When events, circumstances, or even the flow of thoughts isn't going our way, we tend to resist them in ways disproportionate to what is appropriate.

What happens in the brain when we resist? As with attachment, the experience of resistance corresponds to a distinctive pattern of activation in the brain. When we shift from attachment to resistance, the pattern of activation in the brain shifts from the left to the right frontal region of the brain—the region associated with fear and avoidance.[11]

This pattern of avoidance once played an essential role in human survival.[12] It helped us elude hungry and poisonous animals, hostile weather, and other forces of nature that posed an imminent threat to our survival. But in the modern world, much of what we resist poses no actual threat to our survival. Worries about gaining weight, aging, or professional failure—these sources of resistance don't signal impending death. And yet it often feels as if our life is on the line because these forms of resistance activate the very same neural structures as life-threatening emergencies.

Moving the Set Point

Albert Einstein is said to have declared, "We cannot solve our problems with the same thinking we used when we created them." This is a perfect description of the problem we face when trying to shift our happiness set point.

In striving toward a happier life and higher set point, we find it natural to resort to habits of judgment, attachment, and resistance. The paradox is that these are the very forces that establish and hold the set point in place. If we judge our current state as "bad," attach to happiness, or resist negative thoughts and emotions, we end up further from the goal of living a happier life. Psychiatrist Jeanne Talbot explains: "the more we try to avoid thinking/feeling what is really troubling us, the worse it gets."[13] Trying to attain happiness by judging, attaching, and resisting is like fighting to escape from a pit of quicksand: the harder you struggle, the deeper you sink.

Thankfully, there is an alternative strategy—one that you will learn throughout the course of this program. Using the Train Stage practices, we learn to become more aware of these powerful habits of the mind and loosen the grip of this biological machinery. If we do not develop this awareness, these three set point forces tend to run the show. We get anxious, irritated, and reactive without knowing why. Once we begin to see these forces at work, everything changes. We now have a choice—react according to the preprogrammed instincts of our prehistoric past or create new habits of wellbeing and, in so doing, open ourselves up to new possibilities.

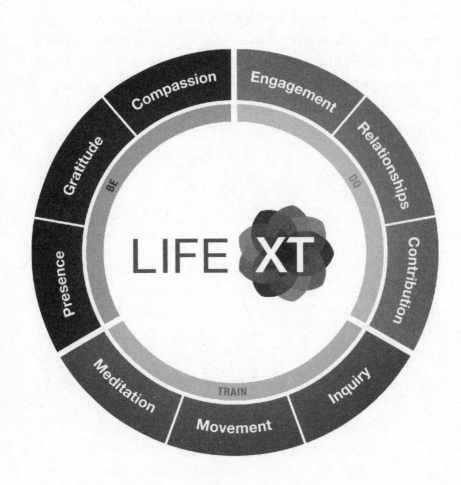

STAGE 1: TRAIN

The Foundation of Wellbeing

The experience of intense physical pain rarely leads to radical scientific breakthroughs. But that's exactly what happened to Richard Davidson on a hot August day in India.

At the time, Davidson was a graduate student in psychology at Harvard. Just a few months earlier, he had convinced the National Science Foundation to fund a trip to Sri Lanka and India.

His trip had a somewhat unorthodox purpose: to dive deeply into the practice of meditation. He told the grant committee that his intention was to study the "relationship between meditation and attention, and between meditation and emotion," and that the only way to properly understand this practice would be to experience it firsthand.[1]

The committee agreed. Several months later, Davidson found himself at a retreat center in India run by a Burmese-born teacher named Goenka.[2] Goenka's meditation technique, called *vipassana*, involved focusing the mind on sensations in the body. As Davidson explains, "We were to slowly and deliberately direct our attention to different parts of our bodies in turn—to what the tips of our noses were feeling, the different temperatures of the air we inhaled and exhaled, how our leg bones felt against the floor."[3]

For the next ten days, Davidson and his fiancée spent roughly fourteen hours a day alternating between walking and sitting meditation. Aches and pains arose, but each time this happened, the retreat participants were instructed to return to the practice: to adopt an attitude of nonjudgmental awareness toward even the most uncomfortable sensations.

After more than a hundred hours spent meditating, Davidson had a breakthrough, an insight that would change the field of neuroscience and psychology. As Davidson recalls:

> *Goenka taught that vipassana meditation offered a path to enlightenment and the eradication of suffering, but over the course of my hundred-plus hours of silent meditation I became convinced that it also had enormous, untapped potential for psychology and neuroscience. I had directly experienced a tectonic change in how I perceived the world, shaking off the concept of pain as if it were no more than a speck of lint on my shirt, and cultivating a deep and lasting sense of contentment in the moment. As a scientist, I had no doubt that what had occurred involved a change in my brain.*[4]

Fast-forward forty years—Davidson has now become the preeminent researcher in the study of the beneficial effects of meditation on the brain.

His body of work has confirmed his post-retreat intuition in 1974: *Happiness is a skill that can be trained.* "We think of happiness like a skill—no different from learning to play music or golf," says Davidson. "We all come into the world with a certain propensity for happiness, but just like any other propensity, to reach very high levels, it needs to be nurtured."[5]

The Train Stage

The Train Stage is the first and most important stage of the LIFE XT program. The three practices in this stage aim to build the mental and physical foundation of habits that cultivate well-being.

The Three Train Stage Practices

1. *Meditation.* Training the mind to enhance focus and awareness of each moment
2. *Movement.* Enhancing physical and emotional health through daily exercise
3. *Inquiry.* Questioning the stressful thoughts that arise from judgment, attachment, and resistance

---

Unlike the Be and Do Stages that follow, these first three practices of the Train Stage require you to set aside a small amount of time: ten minutes a day for Meditation, thirty minutes three times a week for Movement, and a few minutes each day for Inquiry. You will soon see that the time and effort is well spent—these are the most efficient and powerful practices for unwinding the forces of the set point and creating a new set of habits in the brain and body.

These three practices can change your life—they certainly changed ours—but first they must become habits. Creating these new *habits* is at the core of the entire LIFE XT program.

Rewiring the Brain for Wellbeing

Julia wakes up each morning to a deluge of stressful thoughts about the day ahead. The moment she opens her eyes, she reaches for her iPhone to scan the long list of to-dos piling up in her inbox. Already overwhelmed, she spends the next thirty minutes distracting herself by watching the morning news and reading the latest blog posts on a range of light topics from entertainment to sports. Not surprisingly, the rest of Julia's day matches her morning: It's stressful, it's hard, and she's relieved when it's over.

Derek wakes up with a similar torrent of stressful thoughts. But instead of opening the email program on his iPhone, he questions a stressful thought using the Inquiry practice, and spends the next ten minutes practicing mindfulness meditation. He goes on a short run before showering and getting ready for work. By the time Derek walks into the office, his body feels refreshed and energized, his mind open and awake. Like Julia, the rest of his day matches his morning: It's productive, stimulating, and engaging.

The moral of these two stories? Good practices lead to good habits. Good habits form the foundation of wellbeing.

This insight isn't new. Aristotle, who built an entire system of ethics around the goal of happiness, used the word *ethos* to describe habits or customs. In *The Nicomachean Ethics*, he tells us that "moral goodness . . . is the result of habit."[6]

The nineteenth-century American psychologist William James also understood that we need habits. Without them, we couldn't bathe, get dressed, or find our way to the grocery store. "Habit," he observed, "simplifies our movements, makes them accurate, and diminishes fatigue."[7]

Habits work to increase efficiency in the brain and body. They allow us to go on autopilot while completing so-called mindless tasks: washing the dishes, walking down a flight of stairs, or tying our shoes. Think of a life without habits—a life spent relearning these mundane tasks over and over. Instead of effortlessly bounding up the stairs, you would have to learn how each time. Even a short jaunt in the car would generate the white-knuckled anxiety of a sixteen-year-old's driving test. Life would be slow, frustrating, and vastly inefficient.

Habits grease the wheels of life, but the efficiency of habit comes at a price. By making our actions instinctive, even mindless, habits sometimes take away our conscious power to choose and can limit our options.

Take so-called bad habits. Most of us have some habitual vice: it might be eating sugary foods, smoking, drinking, watching too much TV, or twice-daily Starbucks runs. We all know what it feels like to be drawn to something out of habit. We know how easy it is to devour a bag of potato chips without ever *choosing* to do so. In these situations, the "efficiency" of habit overcomes our capacity to choose. The brain switches to autopilot, with our bad habit at the controls.

In subtle, seemingly innocuous ways, this happens all day long. We get up, take a shower, and drive to work along the exact same route, day after day. It's certainly efficient, but this ingrained chain of habits can also make change daunting.

Enter William James's big idea. While our habits often control us, by exerting conscious choice, we can learn how to control them. Like today's neuroscientists, James viewed our habits as *plastic,* malleable. In his words, "*Plasticity*, then, in the widest sense of the word, means weak enough to yield to an influence, but strong enough not to yield all at once."[8] In other words, we can't change all of our habits overnight, but through conscious practice, we can slowly rewire the system with new, more productive habits.

Think of habits like superhighways in our brains. Without awareness, our actions will quickly follow the high-speed route of habit. But through practice, we can exit the freeway—we can drive on the smaller, less efficient side roads. And the more we drive on these side roads, the wider and more traversable they become and the easier it becomes to turn off the superhighway of destructive habits.

The key is awareness, noticing. This is where change starts. When we become aware of our habits, we can now choose whether to follow our usually unconscious conditioning or chart a new pathway of habit. "My experience," James insisted, "is what I agree to attend to. Only those items which I notice shape my mind."[9]

This idea of awareness or noticing lies at the core of LIFE XT. In each of the nine practices, you will learn this essential skill. By learning to direct your attention, you will begin to "shape" your mind and develop habits that will "shape" your life (for more on the science of forming habits, see Appendix 1).

The idea that we can use our attention to train the habits of wellbeing is no longer just a philosophical premise. When James wrote "Habit" in 1890, he foreshadowed what is now one of the hottest areas of neuroscience research: *neuroplasticity*. Using fMRI scans and other imaging techniques, we now have clear empirical evidence to support James's theory: It is indeed possible to train the brain the same way athletes train their bodies.

Neuroplasticity is a game changer. For hundreds of years, scientists assumed that once we reached adulthood, the structures of the brain and nervous system were fixed. The brain, they thought, was like *plaster*—pliable at first but hardening over time. As psychiatrist Norman Doidge explains, "The common wisdom was that after childhood the brain changed only when it began the long process of decline . . . Since the brain could not change, human nature, which emerges from it, seemed necessarily fixed and unalterable as well."[10]

Today, driven by scientific discovery, a new, more optimistic picture has emerged. The brain is less like plaster and more like plastic—it can be changed and transformed in previously unimaginable ways. "The brain," Davidson explains, "has . . . the ability to change its structure and patterns of activity in significant ways not only in childhood . . . but also in adulthood and throughout life."[11]

The exciting discovery that "neurons that fire together, wire together,"[12] dates back to the pioneering work of psychologist Donald Hebb in the late 1940s.[13] By shifting our habitual thought patterns and behaviors, we activate and establish new neural structures in the brain. And by activating these structures again and again, we rewire the brain to create a new set of habits.

Jill Bolte Taylor expresses the difference between habitual thought and intentional thought like this:

> *Your body is the life force power of some fifty trillion molecular geniuses. You alone choose moment by moment who and how you want to be in the world. I encourage you to pay attention to what is going on in your brain. Own your power and show up in your life.*[14]

Taylor touches on one of the primary themes running throughout *Start Here*: the idea that from one moment to the next we choose how to direct our attention. We can choose to let the ordinary habits of the mind fly the plane, so that stress and tension take us to our usual destination. Or we can choose to redirect our attention—to train our mind to experience a more optimal state of wellbeing.

PRACTICE 1: MEDITATION

"I have been meditating for two years now, and it's the best thing I have ever done to help bring more creativity, positive energy, and peace to my life. When I'm tired, stressed, anxious or depressed, I meditate, and it clears my mind, and makes me feel relaxed and happier. I have shared the meditation experience with my friends, and recommend it to everyone I know."[1]

These aren't the words of a Buddhist monk or a guru. These are the words of the American pop icon Katy Perry.

She is not alone. Oprah, Al Gore, Tina Turner, Dan Harris, Congressman Tim Ryan, Russell Simmons, and Angelina Jolie all meditate. When Oprah introduced meditation into her company, the results were, in her words, "awesome: Better sleep. Improved relationships with spouses, children, and coworkers. Some people who once suffered migraines don't anymore. Greater productivity and creativity all around."[2]

Meditation is considered mainstream now, but it wasn't always this way. Fifty years ago, this ancient practice was positioned at the fringes of popular culture. To most people in the West, meditation seemed foreign, exotic, and strange.

The scientific community shared this suspicion of meditation. Davidson, who devoted his career to researching the effect of contemplative practices on the brain, described himself during this period as a "closeted" meditator. In fact, following the publication of

Davidson's first article on meditation, a senior professor cautioned, "Richie, if you wish to have a successful career in science, this is not a very good way to begin."[3]

Fast-forward half a century, and meditation now occupies a very different place in science and popular culture. At technology companies like Google, mindfulness meditation has become a central practice for boosting productivity, reducing workplace drama, and sparking creativity. Even NFL teams like the Seattle Seahawks have begun using meditation as a tool to enhance performance on the field.[4]

This ancient practice has also become increasingly common in the medical community. Following the pathbreaking work of Jon Kabat-Zinn at the University of Massachusetts Medical School, many hospitals and treatment centers now offer classes on mindfulness and meditation. Some doctors prescribe meditation for conditions like anxiety, depression, insomnia, addiction, and pain management.

And within the scientific community, the meditation research of Davidson and others is no longer viewed with disdain. Instead, this research has added significantly to the rapidly growing scientific literature on neuroplasticity, the amazing ability of the human brain to keep learning, growing, and changing.

The science is now clear. Meditation changes the very structure of the brain, reducing stress and promoting overall wellbeing. Because of the overwhelming body of evidence to support the benefits of meditation, this is where LIFE XT begins.

The Mind of a Monk

Meet Matthieu Ricard, a Buddhist monk whose extraordinary brain gives us a window into how meditation works. Born the son

of a French philosopher, Matthieu grew up in the artistic and intellectual circles of Paris, immersed in Western culture.[5]

As a young man, Matthieu had a passion for science and earned
a PhD in cell genetics at France's prestigious Institut Pasteur. But
five years after an initial visit to India, in 1967, he left Europe for
an extended stay in Asia. There he was transformed from emerging
scientist to Buddhist monk. For the next few decades Matthieu
lived in India, Bhutan, Nepal, and Tibet and studied with many
of the great Buddhist masters. Today Matthieu has added to his
résumé accomplished writer and photographer, and through his
humanitarian efforts he has founded more than 120 projects in the
Himalayas. He also serves as the Dalai Lama's French interpreter.

But Matthieu's impressive CV isn't what makes him extraordinary. *It's his brain.*

An fMRI Meditation Retreat

In 2001, Matthieu flew to Madison, Wisconsin, at the invitation of
Richard Davidson, who wanted to explore the effects of meditation
on the brain. Matthieu was an ideal subject.

Most of us envision monks in meditation sitting beneath a tree
with mountains in the background or in some other serene setting. In
Davidson's experiments, however, Matthieu would have to meditate
inside a functional magnetic resonance imaging (fMRI) machine—
a gigantic device with a hollow space in the middle where subjects
are securely strapped to a board and inserted like a turkey on a pan.

Once in the fMRI, Matthieu wouldn't sit in silence or surrounded by the soothing sounds of nature. Instead, a steady cacoph-
ony of mechanical bangs and pops would accompany his attempts
to arrive at a clear and stable state of mind. As anyone who has had

an MRI scan knows, this is hardly the ideal environment for clearing the mind of distractions. Yet, for an experienced meditator like Matthieu, it was easy. After hours inside the machine, he declared, "It's like a mini-retreat!"[6]

The initial results astounded Davidson's team. They first noticed a clear shift in brain activity across different states. Matthieu's brain changed significantly when he shifted from an ordinary to meditative state. Changes also occurred when Matthieu transitioned from one form of meditation to another. The brain imaging showed that the type of meditation—whether one-pointed concentration, compassion meditation, or an "open presence" state of pure awareness—led to very specific changes in the state of various neural networks.

Davidson's team also observed some intriguing activity in Matthieu's prefrontal cortex when he was in a state of meditation. Specifically, researchers noticed a leftward shift in the right-to-left activation ratio in the prefrontal area of his brain. This ratio is one of the most accurate indicators of emotional wellbeing. The more it favors the left side of the brain, the more likely we are to feel happy and emotionally resilient. The more this ratio tilts to the right, the more likely we are to experience anxiety, depression, and other "negative" states.[7]

In Matthieu's brain, the team observed a pronounced shift in left-side prefrontal activation. Meditation appeared to activate brain regions associated with states most of us long to experience more of in life: joy, resilience, and contentment.

A Startling Revelation

Further studies offered even more evidence that Matthieu's many years of meditation training had led to profound changes in the functioning of his brain.

Consider what was perhaps the most unexpected finding—Matthieu's response to what is called the startle test. In Daniel Goleman's description, "The startle reflex involves a cascade of very quick muscle spasms in response to a loud, surprising sound or sudden, jarring sight. The startle reflex starts about two-tenths of a second after hearing the sound and ends around a half second after the sound."[8]

This primitive response originates deep within the brain stem, leading conventional neuroscience to assume that it was impossible to suppress or alter.

Paul Ekman, a leading expert in the psychology of emotion, wanted to see how a lifelong meditator like Matthieu would respond to this test. His team placed sensors on Matthieu's face and body to measure his heart rate, sweat response, and facial expressions. Then they gave Matthieu a ten-second countdown to a booming sound—a loud bang resembling a gunshot.

In all prior studies, subjects were unable either to suppress or to alter their response to such a startling noise. Matthieu, however, was able to do something that science viewed as impossible: He shut down his hardwired reflex by entering into a meditative state.

This stunned Ekman and his team. "When Matthieu tries to suppress the startle reflex," Ekman explained, "it almost disappears. We've never found anyone who can do that. Nor have any other researchers. This is a spectacular accomplishment. We don't have any idea of the anatomy that would allow him to suppress the startle reflex."[9]

Since the groundbreaking research by Davidson and Ekman, researchers have continued to find similar and equally compelling results with studies on long-term meditators from a variety of different spiritual traditions and backgrounds. This growing body of evidence shows that for experienced practitioners, meditation alters the brain in ways previously thought unimaginable. But the benefits of meditation aren't limited to monks and lamas who have mastered the practice. Even if you have never meditated before, with regular practice you can begin experiencing these benefits in a matter of weeks.

WHAT IT IS

The practice of LIFE XT starts with Meditation, which has a rich history, appearing in many of the world's spiritual traditions, and an astonishing body of scientific evidence to validate its benefits.

Yet even with its recent surge in popularity and scientific interest, for many people, meditation still seems mystical and weird. For those who are interested in this practice, the sheer number of different meditation approaches and techniques can seem overwhelming. And for some, the idea of sitting on a cushion, "doing nothing," sounds more like torture than a path to serenity.

Matt, a participant in one of the first LIFE XT programs, at a digital advertising agency in Chicago, explains:

> *I will try anything once, but I admit that I went into mediation with a slightly closed and super-cluttered mind. As an athlete with a ton of energy who loves fast-paced activities, sitting quietly was never something I enjoyed or excelled at. After a couple of sessions, though, I was hooked. I still have a lot to learn and need to continue to practice, but with a full-time job, a toddler, and a three-hour commute, meditation has given me a powerful new way to focus my mind and tackle the day ahead. Throughout my day, I'm able to do more and stay more relaxed and calm while I'm doing it.*

Like Matt, you may be new to meditation or initially feel turned off by the prospect of sitting still with absolutely nothing to do. On its surface, meditation may seem too simple to do any good or too complicated to begin. But these interpretations overlook the essence of the practice. At its core, meditation consists of a family of practices that train the mind to cultivate an awareness of the present moment and to deal more effectively with negative thoughts and emotions. The key is to become more familiar with the movements of the mind.

It's important to point out that mediation does not take any single form. Instead, *meditation* is a term that describes an array of mental practices designed to cultivate wellbeing. Most of these practices fall within three broad categories:

- *Focused-attention meditation.* The aim here is to train the mind's capacity for concentration and awareness of the present moment by focusing on a single point of attention (such as the breath). If you are new to meditation, this is a good place to begin.

- *Mindfulness or open monitoring meditation.* Rather than focusing on a specific object of attention, in this form of meditation you keep your field of awareness open, allowing you to simply witness or observe and thereby become less reactive to thoughts, emotions, and sensory experiences. This is a more advanced practice, as it requires a certain level of mental stability to watch thoughts, emotions, and sensations move through the mind without getting hooked by them.

- *Compassion or loving-kindness meditation.* The aim of this practice is to cultivate deep compassion for all beings, starting with oneself and then extending compassion to friends and family, to people you find difficult, and eventually to all beings.[10] You will learn this practice in the Compassion chapter.

In LIFE XT, you will begin by practicing a form of focused-attention meditation. This practice will enable you to experience three primary benefits:

- First, your meditation practice will help you train your mind for increased emotional fitness. Meditation is to the mind what aerobic exercise is to the body. Just as running improves cardiovascular function, meditation trains the mind in ways that enhance mood, emotional resiliency, and even immune system function.

- Second, this meditation practice will develop your ability to focus. While the mind often wanders involuntarily from thought to thought, you will build your capacity to cut through these mental distractions and sustain your attention for longer periods, leading to greater productivity and improved performance in all areas of life.

- Finally, a focused meditation practice will cultivate a special kind of awareness—an awareness of the present moment. In meditation, Matthieu explained to us, "One remains in a state of vivid, undistracted awareness that not only is fully aware of the freshness of the present moment but is also endowed with a much clearer appreciation of past events and future possibilities."[11]

WHY IT WORKS

Many traditions offer detailed descriptions of the power of meditation going back thousands of years. From Hindus and Buddhists to the ancient Greeks and early Christian fathers, thinkers throughout the ages have seen meditation as a core practice in a spiritual or philosophical life. According to many spiritual texts, meditation offers a way to create sacred moments in the midst of our ordinarily profane day-to-day lives. Meditation helps us unify the everyday with the divine. Many of these texts also point to the powerful emotional and mental benefits of the practice: Meditation, we are told, makes us more focused, emotionally stable, and present to each moment.

The most extensive descriptions of meditation and its benefits are found in Eastern thought. In the classic Hindu text, the Bhagavad Gita, for instance, meditation is described as a technique that delivers a wide range of benefits: "When the mind has become serene by the practice of meditation," it is "unshaken even by the deepest sorrow." [12]

The Dhammapada, a core text of the Buddhist tradition, describes the untrained mind as "a fish hooked and left on the sand [that] thrashes about in agony." It goes on to say, "Hard it is to train the mind, which goes where it likes and does what it wants. But a trained mind brings health and happiness." [13] Long before the invention of the fMRI, the Buddha taught that a focused mind enhanced all aspects of our lives.

Western spiritual traditions also point toward the importance of this practice. In Psalm 46, for instance, we are told to "be still, and know that I am God." Likewise, in Psalm 4, we are told to "meditate within your heart on your bed." These passages show the connection between finding stillness in the mind and communing with the divine.

Like spiritual traditions, Western philosophy also emphasizes the importance of meditative practice. The Stoic and Epicurean schools of ancient Greece both viewed philosophy not as a detached practice of reading and writing but as an "exercise" of reason in which meditation played a central role in life.[14] Marcus Aurelius beautifully captures the Stoic perspective: "You have the power to strip away many superfluous troubles located wholly in your judgment, and to possess a large room for yourself embracing in thought the whole cosmos."[15]

As in many ancient reflections on meditation, here we see references to two kinds of benefits: the practical and the mystical. Meditation allows us to strip away the stress-inducing power of judgment, and it allows us to embrace the whole cosmos. For some, the practical benefits for wellbeing more than justify the time and effort required to start a regular meditation practice. For others, meditation is about both optimizing wellbeing and growing spiritually. It doesn't really matter which you choose. Both approaches—the secular and the spiritual—have the power to change your life in profound ways.

Meditation in our Modern Lives

Matthieu Ricard is a kind of Michael Jordan of meditation. To be considered a long-term meditator like Matthieu, you would have to meditate for upwards of ten thousand hours (at an hour a day, that would take twenty-seven years). "Most people," says Davidson, "with families, jobs and other claims on their time know they will never meditate that much in their lives."[16]

So what benefits does meditation offer those of us with kids, jobs, and other life commitments, and how much meditation do we need to reap these benefits?

To address this question, Davidson's team shifted from studying monks to studying everyday people with no prior training in meditation. Davidson teamed up with Jon Kabat-Zinn, a pioneer in the practical application of meditation. At the University of Massachusetts Medical School in Worcester, he created an eight-week course called Mindfulness-Based Stress Reduction—a course that trains participants in basic "awareness" skills to help them manage stress and acute pain. The course consists of weekly two-and-a-half-hour sessions, forty-five minutes of daily practice, and a one-day retreat.

Davidson's team selected two groups of volunteers from a local biotech company. The first group consisted of "meditators" who would take Kabat-Zinn's eight-week course. The second group consisted of people who were told they were on a "wait list" and received no meditation training. The team measured brain electrical activity of participants in both groups before and after the study.[17]

Davidson's findings showed a clear link between meditation and emotional wellbeing. Anxiety symptoms in the meditation group fell by 12 percent, while anxiety increased in the control group.[18] In the first group, researchers also found a shift toward more left-side activation, an indicator of increased resiliency and emotional wellbeing. Davidson observes, "Compared with what it had been before the course, the level of left-side activation had tripled after four months. The 'wait list' control group actually had less left-side activation."[19]

Meditation, it appeared, changed the brain of these participants. But this study offered one other unexpected insight. At the end of the meditation course, Davidson's team wanted to examine the effects of meditation on the immune system. So they gave participants in both groups a flu shot. They then measured the level of antibodies produced in response to the shot. They found that the levels of antibodies to the vaccine in meditation group participants were 5 percent higher than the other group's levels.[20] Meditation, it appeared, didn't just change the brain; it also changed the body by enhancing participants' immune systems.

Davidson's groundbreaking research both on monks and on ordinary people marked the beginning of an explosion of scientific interest in the practice. In addition to Davidson's early findings, a growing body of research shows that meditation delivers additional compelling benefits key to our performance in most life activities and our overall functioning, including:

- *Increased focus.* Meditation activates additional circuits in the brain that allow for sharper and more efficient concentration.[21]
- *Decreased mind wandering.* Meditation reduces moments when our attention wanders away from what is happening here and now.[22]
- *Enhanced pain tolerance.* After five months of meditation practice, subjects' response to pain in the thalamus decreased by 40 to 50 percent.[23]
- *Slower mental aging.* As we age, the density of gray matter decreases. But meditation appears to counteract this effect by increasing the density of gray matter in the brain, making the brain more facile in old age.[24]

Science tells us *meditation changes the brain.* We have experienced these benefits firsthand and have watched as our clients have changed their lives through simply meditating for a few minutes each day. If you have yet to start a regular practice, we encourage you to experience these benefits for yourself. To not meditate is to miss out on a more focused, productive, happy life, with less stress.

HOW TO DEVELOP THIS SKILL

Follow your breath.

This is the basic LIFE XT Meditation practice. In this practice, the breath anchors the mind. It's the most efficient way to stay in the present moment and keep your mind from wandering.

Here's how to get started. Sit upright—in a chair or on a cushion on the floor—with your spine straight. Place your attention on your breathing. The goal here isn't to focus on *thoughts* about your breath, such as *My breath is too tight* or *Am I breathing right?* The goal is to take your attention deeper—to the embodied sensation of breath: the physical sensations that arise with each new inhalation and exhalation. Notice the sensation of the breath entering and exiting through the nose. Notice the sensation of your abdomen moving in and out, your lungs moving air in and out.

Try it right now. Start with just thirty seconds of placing your attention on the sensations that arise with each inhalation and exhalation.

Don't be surprised if, after even just one breath, your mind starts to wander. This is normal and to be expected. Even the most experienced meditators find their minds wandering to thoughts about delicious french fries, that amazing person they just met, grocery lists, or potential calamities. Meditation isn't about repressing these thoughts. It's about learning to notice them without judgment and then come back, again and again, to the breath.

So when your mind wanders, notice that the mind is thinking. You can even label this mental activity *thinking*. Then come back to the breath.

Meditation is that simple. Focus on the breath and bring the mind back when it wanders. Sounds easy, right? In theory, yes. But in practice, your mind will make things much more complicated. So here are some tips for navigating these bumps in the road and making the most of your meditation practice.

Make It a Habit

Frequency is more important than duration—that is, it's better to meditate for ten minutes a day than to meditate for a single two-hour stretch once a week. As Matthieu puts it, "If we engage repeatedly in a new activity or train a new skill, modifications in the neuronal system of the brain can be observed within a month. It is essential, therefore, to meditate regularly."[25] In LIFE XT, meditation is a daily practice. Carve out time each day, even if it's only a few minutes (for more on how to form habits, see Appendix 1, Habit Formation).

Be Realistic

One of the most frequently asked questions about meditation is *How long do I need to meditate each day to experience the benefits?* There is no single answer to this question. In Davidson's study, subjects participated in forty-five to sixty minutes of mindfulness stress reduction practices each day.[26] Other studies, however, have shown radical changes in brain activation arising from thirty minutes of meditation.[27] In LIFE XT, we recommend that you start with what you can realistically do each day. It could be ten minutes or even five minutes a day. Then, as you progress, you can increase your practice time. It's also important to remember that quality is better than quantity. Spending five minutes in a state of deep concentration is better than a distracted and scattered half hour.

Choose the Right Time and Place

While many people find that meditation works best first thing in the morning, others prefer the afternoon or the evening. The key is to avoid times when you know you will be distracted: Choosing to meditate in the middle of the night when your thoughts are racing is a recipe for meditative failure. Where you meditate is also important. Find a place to meditate that is free from distractions. It might be a corner of your bedroom or a quiet spot in your yard.

Set an Intention

Decide on an inner virtue you aim to cultivate—an *intention*—every time you sit to meditate. It might be to relax. It might just be to sit without getting up for ten minutes.

Adopt a Right Posture

You don't need to sit in a full lotus position with your feet tucked on top of each thigh to meditate. You can sit cross-legged or simply sit on the edge of a chair. The key is to keep your spine erect. Shunryu Suzuki, perhaps the most well-known twentieth-century Zen master, puts it this way: "Keep your spine straight. Your ears and shoulders should be on one vertical line. Relax your shoulders, and push up towards the ceiling with the back of your head."[28] Posture is equally important for overcoming sleepiness. If you slump, your mind will reflect your withdrawn posture. But if you have what Suzuki calls right posture, "you have the right state of mind."

Practice Concentration

The essence of the practice is to direct your attention toward the breath and bring it back each time it drifts. Of course, that is often easier said than done. It requires what Matthieu calls "vigilance": "Whenever you notice that your mind has wandered off, bring it back to the object of meditation."[29] It is this practice of concentration that serves to rewire the brain. The more you direct your awareness toward a single object, the more you create and reinforce new neural pathways.

Don't Judge

When you first start meditating, you will likely notice that your mind churns out a near-constant stream of thoughts. As we have seen, the forces of the mind's set point tend to divide thoughts into the categories of "good" and "bad" or try to resist and stop thinking altogether. In meditation, however, the goal is to cultivate a non-judgmental awareness—to simply sit as the witness, watching as thoughts float in and out of consciousness. Suzuki writes that "If something comes into your mind, let it come in, and let it go out . . . It appears as if something comes from outside your mind, but actually it is only the waves of your mind, and if you are not bothered by the waves, gradually they will become calmer and calmer."[30] As you begin to explore meditation, you will likely find your mind slipping into judgment. You might even start judging yourself to be a "bad meditator." Catch yourself when that happens and open up to the idea that there are no good or bad thoughts. Stay present with the judgments that arise and the sensations in the body that accompany them. Watch them come; watch them go.[31]

Habit 1: Meditation

How to do it: The goal is to make a habit of meditation. So first identify a convenient time and place. As you sit down to meditate, make a brief intention and then begin the practice of mindfully following the breath. You can either set a timer or use one of the guided meditations available at www.LIFE-XT.com. If you are new to meditation, we recommend that you work up to 10 minutes per day using this schedule:

- Days 1 and 2:   3 minutes
- Days 3 and 4:   5 minutes
- Days 5 and 6:   7 minutes
- Day 7:   10 minutes

When you are done with your daily meditation, see if you can take this experience with you into the rest of your day. For more tips and practice strategies, refer to the chapter "How to Practice Life Cross Training" at the back of the book.

Common Meditation Roadblocks

As you begin to meditate, you may run into a few of these common meditation roadblocks:

- *Sleepiness.* Fighting the urge to fall asleep
- *Agitation.* Experiencing anger or frustration
- *Doubt.* Worrying that you aren't doing it right
- *Fear.* Feeling afraid of facing uncomfortable thoughts or sensations

- *Boredom.* Yearning for a different, more exciting or stimulating experience

If you experience any of these roadblocks, good news: You are normal. The key to overcoming each roadblock is the same. Calmly acknowledge and welcome the sleepiness, agitation, doubt, fear, or boredom, and then return your focus to your breathing.

In time, you will learn to be with whatever rises in the mind. This skill will make you less reactive to the ups and downs caused by external circumstances in your life. It will establish a strong foundation upon which to practice the other eight LIFE XT practices. All of these practices are bolstered by the learned skill of focused attention.

The Advanced Practice

Once you have become comfortable with the practice of mindfully following the sensations of the breath and have done it consistently for several months, you can begin to explore a more advanced variation called *open monitoring* or *open awareness meditation.* You might recall that this was the second of the three primary forms of meditation. In this practice, you still use the breath as an anchor. But when thoughts, sensations, sounds, and emotions arise, you will no longer come back immediately to the breath. Instead, you will open the field of awareness and bring all your attention to these various mental phenomena.[32]

To begin, sit in a comfortable seat with a straight spine. Begin with a few minutes of your basic meditation practice, focusing your attention on the sensation of breath. When your mind wanders, bring it back to the sensation of breathing.

Continue with this practice until your mind starts to feel stable. You will know that you have achieved stability by gauging the intensity of your wandering thoughts. If your mind is all over the place—bouncing wildly from thought to thought—then you're not there yet. Return to the breath. When your mind starts to become calmer and you are able to notice more quickly when it wanders, then you are ready to begin the open awareness practice.

Now open the field of awareness. Allow your attention to open beyond the breath to all images, sounds, sensations, or emotions that arise. It's still helpful to place part of your attention on the breath. But if another mental event arises, bring all your attention to it. If, for example, your mind goes to the sound of an airplane flying above your house, bring all of your attention to that sound. Study the soft vibration of the sound: humming, fading, buzzing. Or if your mind goes to a strong sensation of tension in your neck, bring all your awareness to the cluster of sensations that make up the feeling of tension. Study the quality of the sensation: throbbing, gripping, opening. Just be with what is. Don't react. Just watch it. Notice it with equanimity. Tell yourself, *I don't mind what is happening*. As soon as this mental event is no longer predominant, allow your attention to shift to any other mind state in your field of awareness, or return to the sensations of breath.

Joseph Goldstein and Jack Kornfield, two of the most influential contemporary mindfulness teachers, offer a powerful tool for enhancing your practice: "As soon as you become aware that some mind state or emotion or mood is in the mind," they explain, "make a specific note of that particular state of mind, so as not to get lost in it and not to be identified with it."[33] Here are some noting labels you might find useful:

- "Thinking" when thoughts arise
- "Sensing" when sensations arise

- "Hearing" when sounds arise
- "Seeing" when images arise

You can also note emotional states: fear, anger, worry, sadness, etc. In time, this mental noting creates a subtle sense of separation between you and your mind. It will help you remember to watch and witness rather than get hooked by the mind.

Open awareness meditation helps you begin to shift your relationship to the mind. You become the witness or the watcher of mental events. You're no longer a starring actor in the movie of the mind. Instead, you learn to watch the drama unfold, without judgment or identification. This subtle shift will leave you more open, awake, and relaxed in the movie of everyday life.

WHAT TO EXPECT

As you start your meditation practice, it's worth remembering the advice of Jon Kabat-Zinn: "Meditation might be simple, but it certainly isn't always easy."[34] Sitting in silence and watching your breath sounds easy enough. All you have to do is sit there and breathe. But for most of us, the moment we sit, a seemingly endless stream of thoughts and distractions arises. For Eric, it went like this:

My meditation breakthrough happened when I saw that my mind was bored with following my breath. I was more interested in the "things" that I had to think about! My stories had juice in them. So I started telling myself—There will be time for stories after my meditation. I am here to meditate and follow my breath ... follow my breath ...

You may encounter something similar. The breath is simple, and let's face it, sometimes boring. It's so simple that your mind will look for any possible opportunity to explore more "interesting" territory. If you are new to meditation, understanding this paradox is essential. If you think it is supposed to be easy—that your mind will magically stop the moment you sit in meditation—you will likely get discouraged and give up.

In his book *Why Meditate?* Matthieu discusses this initial challenge:

> *When starting to meditate, you might expect that your mind will immediately calm down. Most often, however, just the opposite might happen: it seems that we have more thoughts than before. In fact, your thoughts have not really increased in number; it's just that you have become aware of how numerous they are! Don't be discouraged. It is neither possible nor desirable to try blocking out all thoughts. What matters is to learn how not to be the slave of your own thoughts.*[35]

This is a helpful reminder. Meditation isn't about getting rid of thoughts or dissolving the ego. That's impossible. Thoughts will arise. The mind will wander. You will get distracted. The key is to see these moments as an opportunity rather than a problem. In these moments, you have the opportunity to shift your focus—to notice your mind wandering and bring it back to the breath.

Defining Progress

The meditation teacher Yongey Mingyur Rinpoche, author of the bestselling book *The Joy of Living*, is living proof that mindfulness isn't accidental—it's a trained skill. From the age of six, Mingyur experienced a crippling sense of anxiety, what we in the West would likely call a panic disorder.

When Mingyur first started the practice of meditation, his anxiety didn't go away. "During those early years of meditation," he recalls, "I actually found myself growing more distracted." But Mingyur wasn't getting worse. He tells us "I was simply becoming more *aware* of the constant stream of thoughts and sensations I'd never recognized before."[36]

His experience points to a common pattern. When many people first start meditating, the mind can appear more full of thoughts and distractions than before. But as Mingyur reminds us, this doesn't mean that you are getting worse; it's a positive sign that you are now more aware of your mind. It's like turning on the lights in a messy room—you knew it was dirty before, but now, with the lights on, you are much more aware of the mess.

This experience of increased thought and distraction doesn't happen to everyone. But if it does arise, it's helpful to know that this experience is only temporary. Mingyur, for instance, eventually noticed a shift in his meditation practice that started to loosen these set-point-driven forces of the mind. Through meditation, he recalls, "I began to realize how feeble and transitory the thoughts and emotions that had troubled me for years actually were, and how fixating on small problems had turned them into big ones. Just by sitting quietly and observing how rapidly, and in many ways illogically, my thoughts and emotions came and went . . . I began to see the 'author' beyond them—the infinitely open awareness that is the nature of mind itself."[37]

This experience of feeling less reactive to thoughts, emotions, and sensations is a sign that your practice is progressing. Yet it is important to point out that the whole idea of "progress" in meditation can be misleading. Most of us tend to think of progress as occurring when we have pleasurable experiences, when our thoughts drop away for a short period or when pleasant sensations arise in the body. But the real goal of meditation isn't to get rid of pain and maximize pleasure. True progress is learning to experience fear, sadness, worry, and other painful states, along with more pleasurable states, from a more welcoming, open, and mindful place. In the end, it is the ability to be with whatever is arising—not the fleeting experience of pleasure—that cultivates happiness and wellbeing.

PRACTICE 2: MOVEMENT

Mark had been an athlete in high school and college. He has always won high praise for his athletic abilities, and he took a lot of his confidence and belief in himself from his participation in sports. Soccer, racquetball, and skiing were some of his favorites.

He loved the total immersion and focus that he felt while playing sports, and he carried this skill into his studies and eventually his career, where he quickly achieved success. Mark jumped on the fast track and he began to excel in life. He married the love of his life, they bought a home, and he advanced in his career. By most accounts, life seemed good. Or was it?

I loved giving it my all. But, as with so many of my buddies, work started to take over my life. The demands of taking care of our home and helping my wife with the kids, along with a killer commute, put me on autopilot, and it wasn't long until I began to numb out. I could barely find time to take a shower, much less play sports or even take a walk around the block. I was sitting more than I was moving. I gained weight and felt constant pressure and sadness. Who was this guy, because he sure wasn't me!

One Saturday, a group of friends headed out to play a game of pickup basketball and forced Mark to come along. "Wow! I was winded in minutes and everything in my body ached as I tried to make my 'signature moves.' It hit me like a rock. That was it! Something had to change."

Mark began to carve out time in his schedule to exercise. He booked a racquetball court, starting by just chasing some balls around for an hour a week. He'd also heard about LIFE XT and decided to start the program.

> *I was excited to find movement as the second practice. Boom! I was committed to movement now three times a week for thirty minutes, and my body wanted more. I began to look forward to hitting the court or taking a brisk walk or run, and I felt happy as my muscles began firing and my lungs filled with air. My body was waking up and was tapping my spirit to get into the game. It didn't take much to reconnect with how great movement and exercise made me feel. Now thirty minutes, three times a week is my entry point. I know that regardless of what else is going on, I am going to show up for that promise to myself.*

Mark's story is an example of the profound benefits that arise from something as simple as exercising a few times a week. In fact, research in exercise physiology, neuroscience, and psychiatry shows that the benefits of movement—the act of exercising the body—go far beyond the body. Regular movement also reshapes the mind in numerous ways that promote cognitive performance and emotional fitness.

WHAT IT IS

We use *movement* as an umbrella term for the regular practice of moving the body. All kinds of terms these days describe movement: *working out, exercising, dancing, biking, hiking,* and *cross training.* Don't let yourself get distracted by the words. They all point to a common idea and practice—*moving the body*. Whether we walk, do yoga, run, bike, or swim is unimportant. What matters is that these activities shift us out of what Henry David Thoreau calls the "sedentary life."

An expanding body of research shows that exercising for thirty minutes three times a week has profoundly beneficial effects. It enhances our capacity to learn, makes us more productive, increases our ability to handle stress, elevates our mood, and slows aging.

If exercise were a drug, it would be a miracle pill. And its benefits are dose-dependent. Thirty minutes of brisk walking or running creates a significant shift at the level of mind and body. But so too does thirty seconds of movement. In fact, you can experience this for yourself by running a simple experiment. Choose a time today when you are seated, either at work or at home. Notice your level of energy and aliveness. Then move for thirty seconds. If you are struggling to figure out what to do, try this simple practice. Stand up and then begin rotating your upper body from left to right. Let your arms swing freely in an exaggerated manner so that they flop against your torso. Repeat this twist from left to right, feeling a growing relaxation. Then stop, close your eyes, and notice any change.

WHY IT WORKS

Henry David Thoreau was ahead of his time. He didn't run experiments in psychology. Nor did he have access to the findings of modern neuroscience. And yet this nineteenth-century American philosopher anticipated one of the most cutting-edge insights emerging from these fields: Movement doesn't just keep us fit. It makes us happier.

Thoreau used his own experience as a kind of laboratory for testing the happiness-boosting power of exercise. During his time at

Walden Pond, Thoreau spent each day "sauntering," as he called it. He would walk near the lake or into the countryside. Thoreau's timeless insight wasn't that walking was good for physical health. Even in his day, the physical benefits of exercise were commonly understood.

For Thoreau, the real benefit of walking and other forms of movement went beyond the physical. Movement, he thought, could change us at an even deeper level—*at the level of the mind and spirit.* When we move—especially in nature—he observed, "There will be so much the more air and sunshine in our thoughts."[1]

Thoreau wasn't alone in seeing the vast mental benefits of exercise. Just a few years later, the German philosopher Friedrich Nietzsche landed on a similar idea. He described sedentary life behavior, what he called "ass iduity," as "the real sin against the holy spirit."[2] He also pointed to the same psychological and cognitive shift that Thoreau identified: "Only those thoughts that come by walking have any value," he declared.[3]

Thoreau and Nietzsche weren't the first philosophers to understand the powerful effects of movement on the mind. Plato and Aristotle both viewed physical training as essential to living a philosophical life. In fact, Aristotle's philosophical school—the Lyceum—included exercise grounds and led to his followers being called Peripatetics (those given to walking or moving from place to place).[4] Likewise, the ancient Greek philosopher Zeno, the founder of the Stoic school of philosophy, was said to have spent his days in Athens's Agora, pacing up and down the Stoa Poikile, a long, two-story structure housing shops fronted by a covered walkway—one of the most famous buildings in the city.[5]

For the ancient Greeks, as for Nietzsche and Thoreau, movement was a powerful way to change our inner world by enhancing mood, inspiring creativity, and ultimately serving as a gateway to living a more meaningful life.

• • •

Today we have a vast body of scientific evidence to support the idea that movement cultivates wellbeing. Researchers divide the study of movement into two main categories: *nonaerobic* and *aerobic*. Scientists generally classify yoga, Pilates, and many forms of strength training as nonaerobic forms of movement. These activities offer immense benefits but do not satisfy the core requirement of aerobic exercise— increasing the body's need for oxygen. By contrast, running, cycling, swimming, and hiking all increase the body's demand for oxygen and raise heart rate and respiration above normal resting levels.

Aerobic forms of exercise increase cardiovascular health, lower cholesterol, reduce risk of diabetes, and enhance mood and cognitive functioning. Meanwhile, nonaerobic forms of exercise such as yoga, Pilates, and tai chi offer other benefits. They trigger the relaxation response and enhance mood in ways that decrease mental and physical tension. One type of exercise isn't better than the other. Rather, each is the perfect complement to the other. By combining these two practices, we profit from both the activating qualities of aerobic exercise *and* the strengthening, relaxing, and harmonizing qualities of nonaerobic movement.

Examples of Aerobic Movement	Examples of Nonaerobic Movement
• Walking • Running • Swimming • Dancing • Nordic skiing • Hiking • Cycling • Stair climbing	• Pilates • Yoga • Strength training • Core training • Barre-based workouts • Push-ups and pull-ups • Tai chi • Stretching

How Nonaerobic Movement Affects Wellbeing

There are myriad forms of nonaerobic movement, but let's look at yoga as an example. Over the last thirty years, the popularity of yoga has surged. In *The Science of Yoga*, *New York Times* writer William Broad offers a detailed description of how this ancient practice changes the body and mind. He starts by debunking the many myths about its benefits: Yoga helps you lose weight, increases your aerobic capacity, enhances emotional wellbeing, and so on. Broad shows that the actual science of yoga fails to support some of these claims.

Many people think that yoga promotes weight loss. Yet it turns out that most forms of yoga actually slow the metabolism of the body, which means that, if you eat the same amount of food as you did prior to practicing yoga, you might actually gain weight.[6]

Yoga is also often promoted on the grounds that it improves aerobic capacity. In a Duke University study, however, yoga had virtually no impact on VO2 max capacity (the primary measure of aerobic fitness). Those who engaged in aerobic activities, by contrast, showed increases of around 12 percent. Researchers have arrived at similar findings from studies of a variety of different styles. Hatha yoga, ashtanga, and even power yoga all appear to have a limited ability to increase aerobic capacity.[7]

To many yoga practitioners, these scientific findings may be disappointing. But that's not the end of the story. The most powerful benefits of yoga arise not from its effect on the body alone but from its impact on the relationship between mind and body. In the Duke study, for example, researchers noted a whole host of benefits that straddle the divide between mind and body: enhanced sleep, energy, health, endurance, and flexibility.[8]

One of the most intriguing findings is that yoga corresponds to dramatic increases in gamma-amino butyric acid (GABA), an important neurotransmitter that helps lift mood and prevent depression and anxiety. In a 2007 study, researchers measured the neurotransmitter levels of participants before and after a fifty-five-minute yoga session that included many of the most common yoga poses: inversions, backbends, twists, and sun salutations. They found that the levels of GABA in the brains of beginning yoga students increased by 27 percent after the class. The increases in GABA were even more pronounced in advanced practitioners. One experienced practitioner's GABA levels increased by 47 percent, while another's increased by 80 percent.[9]

A more recent study by John Denninger, a psychiatrist at Harvard Medical School, suggests that yoga also switches on and off genes that control immune function and the stress response. In particular, yoga enhances the expression of genes related to energy metabolism and insulin secretion, while decreasing the expression of genes linked to "inflammatory response and stress-related pathways."[10]

It's one thing to understand that yoga and other nonaerobic practices can increase levels of GABA and suppress harmful gene expression. It's another to feel these powerful effects firsthand. Nate describes his experiences of the physical and mental transformations initiated through the regular practice of yoga:

> At age twenty-seven, I felt like a twentysomething living in the body of an eighty-year-old man. My neck and body were in a state of near-constant pain. My mind swirled with anxiety. I ate constantly. My goal was to simply make it through each day. The tension in my body and mind felt inescapable.
>
> Then one day I joined my wife as she practiced yoga in the liv-

ing room of our apartment. For years, I had teased her about her "downward dogs" and jokingly told her namaste. But after just sixty minutes of yoga that day, I experienced something amazing: I felt myself relax for the first time in years.

I started by practicing yoga a few times a week. Within six months, I was practicing every day. The changes I experienced were gradual but profound. Over the next few years, the daily feeling of pain and tension in my neck slowly subsided. My body felt stronger, my mind steadier. My metabolism even changed, allowing me to return to a more normal way of eating. To say that yoga changed my life feels like an understatement. It changed everything: my posture, my metabolism, my energy level, my resiliency in challenging situations, my ability to focus, my marriage, and the sense of joy I felt to simply be alive.

If you have yet to experiment with yoga or related movement practices, don't take our word for it. We encourage you to test it for yourself.

How Aerobic Movement Affects Wellbeing

If the science supporting nonaerobic movement is promising, the science supporting aerobic forms of movement is astonishing. Research over the last thirty years suggests that moderate and high-intensity aerobic exercise (where your heart rate rises above 65 percent of your maximum heart rate) has profound effects on the brain.

Harvard Medical School psychiatrist John Ratey has painted a detailed picture of the scientifically validated benefits of exercise. Ratey and the work of other researchers shows that aerobic exercise impacts wellbeing on all levels, not just physical health but also how we think, how we age, and how we regulate our emotions.

Scientific evidence points to numerous benefits of aerobic exercise:

- *Enhanced learning.* Exercise enhances learning in three primary ways. As Ratey explains, "First, it optimizes your mindset to improve alertness, attention, and motivation; second, it prepares and encourages nerve cells to bind to one another, which is the cellular basis for logging in new information; and third, it spurs the development of new nerve cells from stem cells in the hippocampus."[11] In fact, enhanced learning capacity reaches its peak directly following exercise. So next time you have a big meeting, presentation, or performance, "going for a short, intense run ... is a smart idea."[12]

- *Greater productivity.* Studies of workplace environments show a strong correlation between exercise and increased productivity. In a 2004 study conducted by researchers at Leeds Metropolitan University in England, 65 percent of workers who exercised reported improvements in interactions with colleagues, time management, and meeting deadlines. And in a study of Northern Gas Company employees, researchers found that those who participated in a corporate exercise program took 80 percent fewer sick days.[13]

- *Increased resiliency to stress.* At one time or another, we've all experienced intense stress. Our hands sweat, our breath shortens, our heart races, and adrenaline courses through our veins. It turns out that regular aerobic exercise acts as a kind of brake on the cascade of hormones our bodies release when under stress.[14] In a world where stress is increasingly hard to escape, the fact that exercise builds our resiliency is good news indeed.

- *Enhanced mood.* For those who struggle with anxiety and depression, aerobic exercise may be just as beneficial as prescription antidepressants. In a 1999 Duke University study, researchers compared the effects of exercise against Zoloft, a popular medication used to treat anxiety and depression. They divided subjects into three groups: an exercise group, a Zoloft group, and a group that did both. The results? Researchers found significant decreases in depression among all three groups, leading James Blumenthal, the head researcher, to conclude that exercise is just as effective as medication in the treatment of depression.[15]

- *Slows aging.* Sooner or later, we all have to deal with the physical and psychological effects of aging. While we can't stop aging, new research shows that by engaging in regular aerobic activity, we can slow the aging process. Exercise reduces blood pressure and strengthens the cardiovascular system; it reduces blood sugar levels, the biggest risk factor for diabetes; it boosts the immune system; and it helps combat the risk of osteoporosis by increasing bone density.[16] The really great news is that exercise not only slows aging in the body but also appears to slow the onset of Alzheimer's disease and dementia. In population studies on dementia, for instance, those who exercise at least twice a week appear to reduce their likelihood of developing dementia by 50 percent.[17]

An impressive and continually expanding body of research shows that regular exercise can transform your inner state. Moving for thirty minutes three times a week will allow you to dissolve stress, enhance your productivity, and help bring the neurochemistry of your brain into balance. It's just a matter of *doing it.*

HOW TO DEVELOP THIS SKILL

The LIFE XT Movement practice is simple. *Move.*

Our program doesn't distinguish between forms of exercise. It doesn't matter whether you walk at a brisk pace, run laps, cycle, ski, play tennis or basketball, or take a dance class. *What matters is that you turn movement into a habit.*

LIFE XT offers a straightforward prescription for movement. If you are just beginning to create a regular exercise program, we recommend:

- Thirty minutes of aerobic exercise, three times per week.
- One nonaerobic workout per week.

This program will help you experience the benefits of both forms of movement. Your three days of aerobic activity will activate the mind and body, building your level of mental and physical fitness. The day of nonaerobic activity will help you avoid injury and maximize the mental benefits of exercise by keeping your body and mind flexible, relaxed, and strong.

If you already have an established exercise program, your weekly routine may far exceed this prescription. In that case, we encourage you to follow a slightly different prescription: *During one of your weekly workouts, do something different.* If you do six aerobic workouts per week, change it up, and once a week, do a nonaerobic workout. If you do all nonaerobic, change it up, and once a week, do something more aerobic. Here again, the goal is to cultivate optimal balance in the body and mind.

Habit 2: Movement

How to do it: Your goal is to make a habit out of movement, so that, like all habits, it takes a minimal amount of willpower and conscious effort to do it. Start by identifying a form of exercise or a mixture of different exercises to begin or add to your routine. Choose something that resonates with you. The possibilities are almost endless: mountain biking, walking, hiking, Zumba, Pilates, yoga, swimming, Nordic skiing, P90X, and on and on. The next step is to set a specific, measurable, and realistic goal. The beginning LIFE XT prescription is to do one form of aerobic exercise for at least thirty minutes three times per week and one nonaerobic workout once a week. For more advanced practitioners, the prescription is to do something different (either aerobic or nonaerobic) once a week. Feel free to set your personal goal above or below this recommended amount. For more tips and practice strategies, refer to the chapter "How to Practice Life Cross Training" at the back of the book.

No matter what your ability level, remember the importance of moderation. While more movement is generally better, too much can create problems. Aerobic exercise, after all, places stress on the body—that's what creates positive change in the mind and body. But if you push too hard too fast, you can overstress the body, which can lead to injury and exhaustion. Nonaerobic practices should also be done in moderation. When it comes to yoga, Pilates, and strength training, too much can result in muscle tears, joint injuries, and other problems.

The key is to listen to your body. If you feel alive and energized after working out, you are in the sweet spot. You can stay there or increase the intensity and time of your workouts gradually. If you feel extreme tension or exhaustion or experience tweaks and minor injuries after your workouts, it's time to dial it back or try something different.

Beyond Exercise: Moments of Movement Throughout the Day

Developing the habit of movement goes beyond simply exercising a few times each week. It's also essential to break out of what scientists call "sedentary behavior" during the other fifteen waking hours of the day.

Scientists used to think that short thirty-minute bursts of exercise were all that mattered—that your activity level during the other hours of the day had no significant impact on wellbeing. But recent findings show that movement, or lack thereof, during our time at work, at home, and in the car has profound effects on health and wellbeing. This research has led some to suggest that "sitting is the new smoking" and surfaced in a *Time* magazine article entitled "Sitting Is Killing You." [18]

In a study of 17,000 Canadians, researchers found a shocking correlation between time spent sitting and increased mortality rates. Even when they controlled for age, smoking, and physical activity levels, researchers found that the individuals who spent the most time sitting were around 50 percent more likely to die during the follow-up period. [19]

Other studies show that such sedentary behavior is strongly correlated with larger waist circumference, higher body mass index, and higher blood sugar levels (a key indicator of one's risk for diabetes).[20]

Why is sedentary behavior so dangerous? First, the more we sit, the more we reduce the energy expenditure of the body. This means that we burn fewer calories and reduce circulation. Second, the more we sit, the more we eat. In studies of TV watching, the number of hours spent sitting correlates with an increase in caloric intake.[21]

The good news is that by taking more breaks, walking more, and sitting less, we can easily reverse these effects (for tips on how to do this, see the chapter "How to Practice Life Cross Training.").

WHAT TO EXPECT

If you already have a consistent movement program, you know firsthand the power of this practice. If you are new to the practice, if it's been a while since you have exercised consistently, or if you are learning a new style of movement, you can expect to experience a few growth stages as you turn this practice into a habit.

The first is the adjustment stage. Your body and mind are driven by habit and are used to a certain level of activity, strain, and energy expenditure. This means that when you start a consistent practice of running, walking briskly, standing more, or doing yoga, the body needs time to adjust. When introducing aerobic forms of exercise, you may tire quickly during the activity or have muscle soreness the next day. When introducing nonaerobic forms of exercise, such as yoga, you may feel stiff or awkward, or you may have difficulty learning how to coordinate your breathing with the postures. The key thing to remember during this first stage is that if you can make it through the learning curve and discomfort of the first few weeks, everything gets easier (for more on this, see Appendix 1, Habit Formation).

Once your body adjusts to a new movement practice (usually after three to six weeks of consistent practice), you will begin the integration stage. At this point, your body will become more accustomed to the activity and you will likely feel less fatigue at the end of each workout. You will also notice a significant decrease in the amount of muscle strain you feel during the days after your workout.

If you stay consistent with your movement practice throughout these two initial stages, you will eventually reach the enjoyment stage. This is where things get interesting. In this stage, exercise ceases to become a chore. In fact, it will quickly become one of the highlights of your day. You will finish running and feel a euphoric "high" throughout the rest of the day. You will finish practicing yoga and feel a deep sense of relaxation and peace that lasts for hours. You will no longer need to focus on how to do the activity or push yourself so hard to do it. Instead, exercise will become increasingly effortless and will often leave you feeling ecstatic.

If you are new to movement or learning a new movement practice, remember that your consistent practice will soon yield the ultimate reward: the blissful physical and emotional enjoyment that comes from moving your body throughout the day. As Thoreau noted, when we move, "there will be so much the more air and sunshine in our thoughts."[22]

PRACTICE 3: INQUIRY

At age forty-three, Byron Katie was about the last person you might expect to become a bestselling author.

At the time, she lived in the Mojave Desert town of Barstow, California, not exactly a mecca for thought leaders on self-improvement. By all accounts, Katie lived a miserable life. She suffered from intense anxiety and suicidal depression, was overweight, and had developed an addiction to codeine and alcohol.[1] Her daughter, Roxann, a sixteen-year-old high school student at the time, described her as "one of the saddest, angriest people I've ever known."[2]

In February 1986, Katie sought help from the only treatment center covered by her insurance—Hope House, a Los Angeles residential treatment center for women with eating disorders. That's when something extraordinary happened. As Katie describes it in her book *A Thousand Names for Joy*:

> *As I lay on the floor of my attic room (I felt too unworthy to sleep in a bed), a cockroach crawled over my foot, and I opened my eyes. For the first time in my life, I was seeing without concepts, without thoughts or an internal story. All my rage, all the thoughts that had been troubling me, my whole world, the whole world was gone.*[3]

The ancient spiritual traditions have many names for this flash of insight. The Buddhist tradition calls it *bodhi:* the enduring state of liberation from suffering. In the West, we tend to use the word *enlightenment.* But Katie describes her insight that day as something simpler but no less profound:

> *I discovered that when I believed my thoughts, I suffered, but that when I didn't believe them, I didn't suffer, and that this is true for every human being. Freedom is as simple as that. I found that suffering is optional. I found a joy within me that has never disappeared.*[4]

Whatever it was that happened on that morning, it changed Katie. When she returned home, her family was in shock. "It was like they dropped off a completely different person," recounted her daughter, Roxann.[5]

Katie now travels the globe helping people question their thoughts and find a sense of freedom. She is the author of several bestselling books, leads retreats and workshops throughout the world, and was dubbed by *Time* magazine "a spiritual innovator for the new millennium."[6]

Katie calls the method of questioning that she discovered on that February morning inquiry, or "The Work." It is the practice you will learn at the end of the chapter—a practice that will enable you to begin releasing the hold of even your most stressful beliefs and stories. By questioning your stressful thoughts, you will reduce stress, anxiety, worry, and unhappiness and begin feeling more free, open, and centered.

Talking to Ourselves

Katie's process of questioning our thoughts has a long and venerated history. In the West, the practice of Inquiry dates back thousands of years, to a shabbily clothed older man with bulging eyes and a potbelly—a man who often stood in the market square questioning his thoughts and those of passersby. Today we would likely dismiss a man like this as "crazy," "weird," or "homeless." He did, in fact, explain to those who asked that he had what he called a *daimonion,* a voice in his head that gave him advice, mostly telling him what *not* to do. "This is something which began for me in childhood," he would explain. "A sort of voice comes, and whenever it comes, it always turns me away from whatever I am about to do."[7]

This man was not a social parasite or a crazy person. His name was Socrates, and he was a man many scholars consider to be the first philosopher.

Socrates was born in Athens in 469 BCE, the son of a stonemason. Instead of following in his father's footsteps, in an abrupt departure from the custom of the time, Socrates devoted his life to learning how to live well.[8]

This unconventional path led Socrates to the city streets. Rather than "hold court" in the houses of the wealthy like the other professors of wisdom, he roamed the city talking to just about anyone who would listen—including himself.[9] Socrates had no school, had no formal method, and wrote no books. But he did have one powerful tool: inquiry. In various ways, he repeatedly asked the question of himself and others, *Is it true?*

Socrates questioned everything—even the gods. One day his good friend asked the oracle at Delphi, "Is anyone wiser than Socrates?" The oracle replied no, implying that Socrates was the wisest person in the land. But Socrates didn't take the god's word for it. He *inquired*.

Socrates approached all the so-called wise men of his day: high-ranking politicians, noblemen, and others reputed for their knowledge. Surely, he thought, they would prove to be wiser than he.[10] In the end, however, he found their "wisdom" to rest on a foundation of beliefs and concepts that crumbled under scrutiny. They knew general things about their trade—how to write a poem or build a house—but when it came to wisdom, he was astonished to find that "they know nothing of what they speak."[11]

All this questioning led Socrates to a profound insight about the nature of wisdom—an insight that sits at the heart of the Inquiry practice. As Socrates put it after questioning one of the most highly regarded statesmen of his day,

I am wiser than this man, for neither of us appears to know anything great and good; but he imagines he knows something, although he knows nothing; whereas I, as I do not know anything, so I do not imagine I do. In this trifling particular, then, I appear to be wiser than he, because I do not imagine I know what I do not know.[12]

Real wisdom, Socrates tells us, doesn't arise from the elaborate beliefs we hold about our lives or the stories we tell ourselves about the world. Real wisdom arises from knowing that you don't know.

This idea is simple and yet radical. Today, after all, most of us live like the "wise men" of Socrates's time. We tell ourselves thousands of unquestioned stories about what we believe to be true about the world. We believe thoughts like *I can't, She/he doesn't love me,* or *I don't have enough* (money, time, love, etc.). We can live our entire lives believing these seemingly certain truths, without ever calling them into question.

What Socrates teaches us is that until we pose a simple question to ourselves—*Is it true?*—we have no way of knowing. Who knows? It might be that all the "problems" you worry about are actually possibilities. It might be that your "defects" are your greatest strengths. It might be that those goals you see as "impossible" are well within reach.

WHAT IT IS

Beneath every stressful emotion sits a thought—a thought that may or may not actually be true. Once you question the validity of the thought, the accompanying stress in the mind and body starts to fall away.

Alex, founder of a professional services firm, talks about experiencing this shift firsthand:

> *I became convinced that a competitor was trying to poach my staff, despite having no evidence that this was the case. I shared my concerns with my brother. Instead of commiserating with me and validating my feelings, my brother asked me, "Do you know that this is true?" This simple question forced me to question my assumptions and, through this, to understand the cascading effect of negativity that holding on to my story generated. Even more important, I realized that this one thought had created a tidal wave of stress, anxiety, and anguish. When I let go of the belief, something amazing happened: The ache in my stomach and worries that kept me sleepless for nights disappeared.*

Alex describes the power of asking *Is it true?* in the midst of a stressful life situation. Try it right now. Identify one stressful thought that you have about another person (spouse, coworker, friend, child, etc.). Now ask yourself, *Is it true?* Your instinct might be to say yes, but sit with it for thirty seconds. Consider the possibility that it might not actually be true.

The practice of Inquiry is a more systematic approach to this exercise—a tool that will help you go even deeper. The power of this practice arises from the fact that our experience of life is shaped by a thick web of interconnected stories and beliefs. We judge ourselves: *I'm too fat. I'm not good enough.* We attach: *Nothing ever turns out right. I need more money.* We resist what is: *It's too cold out. My daughter should listen to me.* These stories and beliefs play in our minds like background music at a restaurant, so familiar that we are no longer conscious of them. But we hear their message anyway.

This web of stories and beliefs is powerful. It is the lens through which we view the world. If you think constantly about gaining weight, you begin to see the world through the lens of calories, workouts, and pants sizes. If you think constantly about making more money, you begin to see the world through the lens of financial reports, status, and envy.

Without calling these stories and beliefs into question, we tend to just assume their truth. *My neighbor is being irrational. My child's soccer coach is unfair. My boss is controlling.* These kinds of everyday stressful beliefs become our holy doctrine. And the more we cling to them, the more we experience stress, anxiety, and unhappiness.

The practice of Inquiry invites us to shift our ordinary way of being in the world. Change starts with the Socratic question, asking *Is it true?* This simple act of questioning the thoughts that shape our reality has the power to unwind the web of beliefs holding the set point in place. It opens our inner world to a new way of being and has a direct impact on our outer world—leading to our living a life with more compassion, ease, and openness to new possibilities.

WHY IT WORKS

Socrates was not alone in detailing how our thinking causes us pain and suffering. Around five hundred years later, the Stoic philosopher Epictetus declared, "We are disturbed not by what happens to us but by our thoughts about what happens."[13] Some fifteen hundred years later, Shakespeare drew a similar connection in Hamlet's dialogue with Rosencrantz: "There is nothing either good or bad, but thinking makes it so."[14]

Historical accounts of inquiry also describe in great detail the paradoxical goal of this practice: learning to know that you don't know. The skeptics of ancient Greece based their entire approach to philosophy on this ideal. *Skepsis* (skepticism) is the Greek word for investigation. At the core of skeptical thought lies the idea of striving to attain "a life without belief"—a life where wellbeing and inner peace arise not through accumulating knowledge but through questioning all that we think we know.[15]

The Zen tradition talks about this ideal of "not-knowing" as aspiring toward "the beginner's mind." "In the beginner's mind," says Shunryu Suzuki, "there are many possibilities; in the expert's mind there are few ... When we have no thought of achievement, no thought of self, we are true beginners. Then we can really learn something."[16] Stephen Mitchell, the acclaimed poet, translator, and anthologist, told us that his teacher, the Zen master Seung Sahn, offered students a similar description of the goal of inquiry. "I have brought just one teaching to America," he insisted, "Don't-know mind. That is all you need to know: Don't know."[17]

Other traditions, such as the Madhyamaka School of Tibetan Buddhism, point to a similar method of attaining this state, what some call "the meat grinder of the mind." To clear out the many illusions of the mind, these teachings recommend questioning everything, even the most basic assumptions we hold about the world.[18]

Whether it is Socrates, Epictetus, or Buddhist traditions, thousands of years of enduring wisdom point to inquiry as an essential tool for loosening the set point forces of the mind. Using different words, each of these philosophies makes a similarly surprising and thought-provoking claim: Wellbeing and inner clarity don't arise from amassing new beliefs and knowledge. This optimal state of being arises from questioning the mind and letting go of what we think we know.

In the language of modern psychology, this Socratic form of questioning is called cognitive behavioral therapy (CBT). CBT has become one of the predominant therapeutic modalities in modern psychology, and its many benefits have been documented by extensive research.[19] This tool dates back to 1955, when the American psychologist Albert Ellis revolutionized the field of psychology by introducing a technique he called rational emotive behavior therapy. Yet Ellis didn't create this approach out of whole cloth. Rather, he discovered it in the pages of the ancients. In his words:

> One of the major influences on my thought at the time was the work of the Greek and Roman Stoic philosophers (e.g., Epicurus [sic], Epictetus, and Marcus Aurelius). They emphasized the primacy of the philosophic causation of psychological disturbances . . . This view was also largely promoted by several ancient Asian philosophers,

especially Confucius, Lao-Tsu, and Gautama Buddha. In essence,
these ancient philosophies . . . became the foundation of rational
emotive behavior therapy.[20]

While Ellis created the first therapeutic protocol for what
would come to be known as cognitive behavioral therapy, Aaron
Beck, professor emeritus at the University of Pennsylvania, was the
first to research the method's effectiveness. At its core, the methods
developed by these two men are based on the idea that humans
have a biological tendency toward unhelpful and often irrational
thinking. Our beliefs about life can quickly fall into the traps of all-
or-nothing thinking, jumping to conclusions, fortune-telling, and
focusing on the negative.[21]

Like ancient forms of inquiry, cognitive behavioral therapy uses
reason as a corrective tool to question the often irrational beliefs
that tend to permeate our thinking. Martin Seligman, one of the
founding fathers of the field of positive psychology, writes in his
book *Learned Optimism* that cognitive behavioral therapy offers
three primary tools for disputing our stressful thoughts:

> *First, you learn to recognize the automatic thoughts flitting through*
> *your consciousness . . . Second, you learn to dispute the automatic*
> *thoughts by marshaling contrary evidence . . . Third, you learn to*
> *make different explanations, called reattributions, and use them to*
> *dispute your automatic thoughts.*[22]

Whether you call it inquiry, not-knowing, beginner's mind,
or cognitive behavioral therapy is unimportant. The power of this
age-old practice arises from its benefits. When you question your
stressful beliefs and stories, you begin to see that these ordinary
mental habits of catastrophizing, fortune-telling, and focusing on

the negative have no real basis in reality. You see that stress often arises from stories made up in the mind.

HOW TO DEVELOP THIS SKILL

Philosophers, psychologists, and spiritual teachers have developed hundreds of techniques for questioning the mind. We have explored many of these tools and found that, for LIFE XT, the approach developed by Byron Katie, the woman discussed at the beginning of this chapter, holds the greatest power to cut through our stressful stories and beliefs.

Inspired by her realization that it is our thoughts—not our circumstances—that make us suffer, she created a simple and yet profound tool for questioning stressful stories. She calls it The Work. You can explore it further both on her website (www.The Work.com) and in two of her books, *Loving What Is* and *A Thousand Names for Joy*.

This is the tool you will use in the Inquiry practice. As with most LIFE XT practices, the first step is noticing. Begin by catching yourself when a particularly stressful set-point-driven thought arises. It might be a judgment, such as the thought that your spouse should do more to support you. It might be an attachment, such as a worry about losing a close relationship with your child as he or she graduates and moves off to college. It might be resistance, such as running away from a potentially huge opportunity because you're afraid you might fail.

We recommend starting with your judgments about others (friends, spouse, family members, coworkers). With practice, you can also begin to use it to question your internal judgments and stories (*I'm not good enough, I'm too fat, I'll never be able to . . .*).

Once you have identified the stressful thought, write down your responses to the following questions:

1. Is it true?
2. Can I absolutely know that it's true?
3. How do I react—what happens—when I believe that thought?
4. Who would I be without the thought?

Take your time in answering these questions. Think of this as a kind of meditation. Rather than rushing through the process, pause for a few moments after asking each question and close your eyes. Let the answers arise in your mind without trying to anticipate them. You may be surprised at what you discover.

Once you have answered the first four questions, you are ready for the final step—what Katie calls the turnaround:

5. Turn the thought around (consider its opposite) and then find at least three specific, genuine examples of how each turnaround is true for you in this situation. For instance, if the stressful story is *My husband doesn't appreciate me,* the turnaround might be *My husband does appreciate me, I don't appreciate myself,* or *I don't appreciate my husband.* If the stressful story is *My mother is controlling,* the turnaround might be, *I'm controlling* or *My mother is not controlling.*[23]

Pause and see what answers emerge. With each turnaround that arises, write down three reasons why it is just as true as, if not truer than, the original thought.

Inquiry Tips

- *Write down your stressful thoughts.* It's tempting to try to do this practice in your mind, but by writing your responses down, you create a subtle sense of distance between yourself and your thoughts.
- *Answer yes or no.* The answer to questions 1 and 2 is one syllable only: *yes* or *no.* Notice when you want to justify or defend by saying *but* or *because.*
- *Do it without a motive.* Katie recommends that you engage in this Socratic form of inquiry from a place of genuine curiosity and a desire to know the truth. When you do The Work with a motive—even a noble one such as saving your marriage or improving your life—your answers may be arising from old solutions that haven't worked. Close your eyes after asking yourself each question and allow the answers to appear in your mind.
- *Stay in the situation.* Identify a specific situation where you experienced the stressful thought. As you ask each question, put yourself back in that situation. Allow your memory of that moment to help you understand how you reacted and see how your experience might have shifted without the thought.

Some people feel overwhelmed at the very thought of questioning their thoughts: *How can I question everything all the time?* Remember that the Inquiry practice isn't about questioning all of your thoughts all the time—that would be impossible. It would be a waste of time to do the work on a thought such as *The table is big* or *The sun will rise tomorrow.* These thoughts don't typically cause any stress. Instead, the goal of inquiry is to question the thoughts that create painful emotional responses. And questioning one stressful thought can unravel many stressful thoughts.

When it comes to thoughts like *My boss is so overbearing*, *I'm never going to get my break in life*, or *I can't feel at peace until . . .*, inquiry offers a powerful antidote. It opens the mind to a new set of possibilities. You begin to experience firsthand the insight that Socrates arrived at after questioning the "wise men" of his day: that true wisdom arises from knowing that you don't know.

Habit 3: Inquiry

How to do it: Start by identifying a stressful thought to question. If you are having trouble or just want a deeper experience of Inquiry, use the Judge Your Neighbor Worksheet (available for free at www.TheWork.com). The worksheet will help you generate a list of stressful thoughts to question. Once you have identified the thought, it's time to begin the process of Inquiry. When asking yourself the four questions and turnaround of The Work, you can write out your responses on index cards or, if you would like a more guided experience, print out the One-Belief-at-a-Time Worksheet (also available for free at www.TheWork.com). The next step is to meditate on and write out your answers to the four questions:

1. Is it true?
2. Can I absolutely know that it's true?
3. How do I react—what happens—when I believe that thought?
4. Who would I be without the thought?

(continued on next page)

The final step is to turn the thought around (consider its opposite) and write down at least three specific, genuine examples of how each turnaround is true for you in this situation. Because stressful thoughts often arise within a web of other stressful thoughts, we also encourage you to experiment with a few deeper dives into The Work in which you spend time questioning each of these stressful thoughts as they arise, in sequence. For more tips and practice strategies for Inquiry, refer to the chapter "How to Practice Life Cross Training" at the back of the book.

In our own lives, we have found Inquiry to be one of the most powerful LIFE XT practices. Eric learned about the power of Inquiry when he started to question his beliefs about his son and then watched how their relationship was radically transformed:

I value kindness, generosity of spirit, and compassion. Several years ago, my son Alex started being overly negative and mean to his siblings, to my wife, Sharon, and to me. Often, our interaction would be something like this:

Me: How did school go today, sweetie?
Alex: Fine—although school sucks.
Me, starting to escalate: Why do you have to be so negative?

Each jab back at Alex served only to intensify this verbal sparring. I would criticize him for being negative, Alex would react defensively and say something out of anger, and that would fire me up even more. It was a vicious circle. I knew something had to change, so I began my own Socratic inquiry. Alex shouldn't be so mean. Is it true? *I asked myself. No, Alex should express himself. Alex should feel safe communicating frustrations at home. And then I turned it around to myself:* I shouldn't be so mean. *The evidence was overwhelming. I was being negative toward Alex. I gave him no breathing room. I jumped on him for even the slightest perceived transgression.* I shouldn't be so negative. *In that instant, two profound shifts occurred: First, I stopped jumping on Alex. I gave him the space to be who he wanted to be.* Let any negativity and meanness roll, Alex, *I thought.* I will greet you with presence, love, and acceptance. *Second, as soon as I stopped being negative, Alex dropped his caustic comments almost immediately. The hugs started up again, as did the warmth and love between us. To this day we have a special relationship, and Alex is one of the most loving people I know.*

The more you inquire, the more you will begin to see the connection between stressful thoughts about others and the way others react to you. Katie explains this connection by saying, "The world is the mirror image of your own mind." What she means is that the world we inhabit mirrors our stressful thoughts and beliefs. Before Inquiry, Eric and Alex mirrored each other, leading to a cycle of negativity. After Inquiry, Eric and Alex still mirrored each other, but when Alex was negative or mean, the stressful thoughts fell away from Eric, leaving space for more love and connection.

WHAT TO EXPECT

In our work with individuals, groups, and organizations, we have found Inquiry to be one of the most transformative life habits—but it is also one of the most challenging. It is challenging because it asks us to let go of what we think we know and approach life with curiosity instead of certainty. Yet its benefits are immense. We have watched our own as well as our clients' stressful thoughts, anxieties, fears, and triggers melt in the face of questioning.

As you start the practice of Inquiry, be on the lookout for the following challenges and roadblocks:

- *Going too fast.* Many people approach Inquiry as though they are writing an email or sending a text. They do it as quickly as possible so they can move on to the next thing. If you catch yourself falling into this trap, consciously slow down. Allow yourself to really sit with each of the questions. Sit with each of the four questions for a few moments before writing out your response.

- *Getting curious.* At the very beginning, engaging in Inquiry requires a leap of faith, letting go of what you think you know. For many people, this can feel strange, even scary. So there is a tendency to resist questioning stressful thoughts. If you encounter this challenge, see if you can get radically curious. See what happens when you allow yourself to question what you think you know.

- *Missing the turnarounds.* When you first start, it can be easy to miss some of the turnarounds, the final step of Inquiry. Stressful beliefs about other people can be turned around in three ways: to the self, to the other, and to the opposite. For instance, the thought *My boss doesn't respect me* can be turned around in the following three ways: (1) To the self—*I don't respect myself.* (2) To the other—*I don't respect my boss.* (3) To the opposite—*My boss* does *respect me.* Try to identify each of these turnarounds, and then list three specific, genuine examples of how they are true.

We have found that the practice of Inquiry develops through a couple of stages. The first is the learning stage. Unlike some LIFE XT practices, which are intuitive and require almost no time to master, Inquiry can take time to learn. At the beginning, you may find it strange to reflect on the thoughts that cause you the most suffering. It may also take some time to become familiar with the four questions and the turnaround. This is a natural part of the learning process, and if you ever get stuck, it's worth visiting Byron Katie's website (www.TheWork.com), which offers a wealth of helpful tools and resources.

Once you learn the technique, you will enter the stage of unwinding your stressful thoughts. During this stage, you will begin to experience a steady change in your thinking. It's a lot like letting the air out of a tire. The air doesn't come out all at once. But if you continue to hold the valve open, the pressure in the tire slowly and steadily drops. Inquiry works in the same way—it's an inner technology for deflating the beliefs and stories that create stress in our lives.

During this stage of unwinding, some people fall into the trap of expecting to be able to get rid of their stressful beliefs. In our experience, this rarely happens. For those who worry about not having enough money, for example, Inquiry is unlikely to eradicate all thoughts about finances. It will, however, change your relationship to these thoughts. They will have less power over you.

As you continue to deepen your practice, you can expect benefits on two levels. First, you will notice a change in the way you experience the world. You will notice that the situations, thoughts, and people who once caused you incredible stress no longer trigger you in the same way.

Additionally, you can expect to see a change in your relationships. When Eric learned to drop his own feeling of negativity toward his son, his son became less negative, and their relationship improved almost instantly. The more you practice Inquiry, the more you can expect similar changes in your relationships. By questioning the thoughts that cause worry, irritation, and resentment toward the people in your life, you open a space for more love, trust, connection, and personal peace.

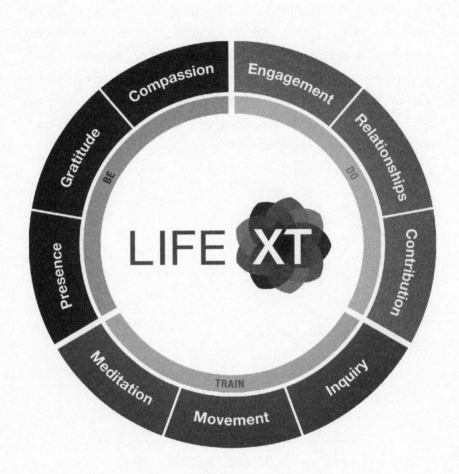

The Practice of Being and Doing

Few people understand winning like basketball legend Bill Russell. He has eleven championship rings, more than any other player in the history of the game—that's six more than Lakers star Kobe Bryant's five, and almost twice as many as the great Michael Jordan's six. But Russell had a winning secret so strange that he could never bring himself to share it with his teammates.

In the heat of competition, he would shift into what he called a "mystical spell"—an altered state of being. "I'd hint around to other players about this feeling," Russell admitted, "but I never talked about it much . . . I felt a little weird about it, and quite private."[1]

In these moments, said Russell, something amazing happened. "That feeling is difficult to describe . . . When it happened I could feel my play rise to a new level. It came rarely, and would last anywhere from five minutes to a whole quarter or more."[2]

In these states, time would begin to expand. "I'd be putting out the maximum effort, straining, coughing up parts of my lungs as we ran, and yet I never felt the pain. The game would move so quickly that every fake, cut and pass would be surprising, and yet nothing could surprise me. It was almost as if we were playing in slow motion."[3]

Not only did everything slow down, but he also started to develop an awareness of how each play would unfold. "During those spells I could almost sense how the next play would develop and where the next shot would be taken."[4]

Most surprising to Russell was the shift out of his usually ultra-competitive mind-set. Rather than playing to win, Russell would play for the sheer joy of this ecstatic experience. "I'd find myself thinking, 'This is it. I want this to keep going,' and I'd actually be rooting for the other team. When other players made spectacular moves, I wanted their shots to go into the bucket; that's how pumped up I'd be."[5]

In this state, winning no longer mattered. "Sometimes the feeling would last all the way to the end of the game, and when that happened I never cared who won."[6]

As an eleven-time NBA champion, Russell had many moments where he felt "moved or joy." And yet, as he puts it, "These were the moments when I had chills pulsing up and down my spine."[7]

When Being Meets Doing

Russell's description of his "mystical spells" offers a window into the experience that emerges from the final two stages of the LIFE XT program: Be and Do. Being is a state of awareness that arises when you wake up to each moment. Doing is about your actions in that state, when you are fully engaged and bringing your greatest possible contribution to the world.

Most books on self-development focus on either being or doing. Books about being speak of the benefits of slowing down, becoming present, and feeling the incredible joy of our aliveness. Books about doing, on the other hand, focus on maximizing productivity, achieving, finding a sense of purpose, and succeeding in work and life. It's easy to focus solely on one or the other of these skills—to think that the key to wellbeing arises from either being *or* doing, but not both.

Some people are prone to falling into the trap of being without doing. Thad, a martial arts instructor and acupuncturist, for example, feels content but sometimes adrift.

I naturally tend much more toward being rather than doing. When my days are open, I tend to lose track of time, easily spending several hours training martial arts in the park, cooking, or socializing with friends. At the same time, it becomes difficult to follow through on the nuts-and-bolts details of my life, such as bookkeeping and work correspondence. On the one hand, I like that I can fully immerse myself in the experience of the moment, but I also find that I start to fall behind on ordinary tasks.

Other people are more apt to fall into the opposite trap: doing without being. Peggy, a high-achieving executive at a health-tech company, describes her experience:

Being productive isn't an issue for me, but being present is. My job at a fast-paced start-up requires me to work long hours, nights, and weekends. I tend to be so productive in my professional environment that I often feel like I can't be truly present and focused on the things I most value—being a wife and mother to two small girls. So when I'm not trying to sneak work in at off times to get it all done, I'm at home giving baths, tucking in the kids, and trying to keep the business of our home in order. The thought that keeps looping through my mind is "There's just not enough time." I want to be successful at work, and I want to be a great mom. But I also realize that to be successful at both, I need to catch my breath and carve out time to simply be.

Both Thad and Peggy feel like something is missing. That's because the path to wellbeing isn't just about learning the art of being *or* doing. It's about learning to combine and balance these two essential parts of life—to train the skill of experiencing the present moment while also engaging in productive activity and bringing your unique gift to the world.

This is what makes Bill Russell's story so extraordinary. We often associate being fully in the present moment as the cessation of doing, as sealing ourselves off from the distractions of the modern world through meditation, long walks, or weekend retreats. But Bill Russell didn't live alone in the woods or spend hours each day in deep meditation. Russell played basketball. He traveled from city to city, playing for hours each night in an arena packed with screaming fans.

Russell didn't stop doing. And yet, in the midst of the madness of playing championship-level basketball, he experienced the awake state of being. He reached the state of present moment awareness described by so many ancient mystics, yogis, and philosophers, not while reciting a mantra or praying but while rebounding, cutting to the basket, and shooting a fadeaway jumper.

The stories of Russell, Thad, and Peggy offer a glimpse into the lesson at the heart of *Start Here*. It's not enough to *be awake*, to passively experience the fullness of each moment. Wellbeing arises from integrating both being and doing into our everyday lives.

The Be and Do Stages

Be and Do are the two integration stages of the LIFE XT program. They represent a departure from the type of practices developed in the Train Stage. In the Be and Do Stages, we shift from daily training to life integration. Unlike Meditation, Movement, and Inquiry, building the final six habits of these stages doesn't require taking time out of life to train. Instead, developing the Be and Do skills simply requires attention.

The goal of the Be practices is to learn to notice when you are lost in the thought stream of the mind and shift your attention back to this moment. The goal of the Do practices is to cut through the internal and external distractions you encounter each day and shift your attention toward engaging more deeply at work, in relationships, and in efforts to contribute to the world.

The ultimate aim of the Be and Do Stages is to integrate the practices of LIFE XT into the moment-to-moment experience of your life.

Stage 2: Be

- *Presence*—experiencing each moment fully as it is
- *Gratitude*—feeling deep appreciation for all aspects of life
- *Compassion*—extending empathy and love to all (including oneself)

Stage 3: Do

- *Engagement*—doing activities that promote the experience of total absorption or "flow"
- *Relationships*—deepening bonds with family, friends, and colleagues
- *Contribution*—merging loving-kindness with acts of generosity

---

Being

Waking Up to Your Life

In each moment, our experience sits somewhere on this spectrum:

ASLEEP	AWAKE	
⟵	⟶	**BEING**
Distracted	Focused	
Worried	Relaxed	
Spaced out	Aware	
Irritated	Accepting	

Your location on the axis of being can change radically from moment to moment. In one instant, you might be awake and aware, gazing into the eyes of your significant other during a romantic dinner. And then in the next, a thought lands: *I forgot to send that email.* This thought spawns another: *I have to submit that report.* And another: *Why didn't my boss copy me on the update she sent around?* And so on. In a fraction of a second, you can go from being awake and aware in the moment to being asleep and distracted.

Look closely at your experience of each moment: How much time do you spend in this sleeping state? When you did the laundry yesterday, when you dropped your kids off at school, when you worked out at the gym—were you fully present? Were you awake to the moment?

If you are like most people, you probably spend the bulk of your time on autopilot, going from one email to another, from one errand to another, from one meeting to another, until finally, at the end of the day, you fall into literal sleep. This is how many of us live our lives.

The goal of the three Being practices—Presence, Gratitude, and

Compassion—is to train the habit of waking up from this ordinary state of mind wandering. These practices help us notice when we have fallen asleep to life and shift by drawing our attention back to one of these three portals to the present moment.

The word *being* might sound mystical to some, but being is simply the experience of what is happening right now. When we live outside the present moment, we easily lose sight of and "fall asleep" to what is here and now. We get lost in a dream populated by thoughts, worries, and desires—past and future. We become so distracted by mind wandering that being fades into the background. Yet it is always there, and we can always come back to it.

Priti, the first corporate mindfulness teacher for LIFE XT, still gets caught in this sleeping state. But she has developed a powerful way of catching herself:

> *My trick is simple:* Beware *of mental "task-listing." All my life, I have been a high achiever, and have done so by creating lists of tasks that I need to accomplish. Over the years, this has transformed into a habit of creating those lists in my mind instead of on paper. Every time this habit kicks in, the result is an immediate departure from the present moment; my mind is anticipating what I have to do later that day, week, month, or even year. Recognizing myself in mental task-listing mode is a clear and vivid reminder that I am not being present. I use it as my cue to shift my attention back to this moment.*

You have probably engaged in something similar to the state of task-listing that Priti describes. It's the experience of *becoming* rather than *being*—constantly looking ahead to the next task, meeting, or email. As University of Chicago neuroscientist John Cacioppo told us,

People spend a lifetime striving to become *something they think they should be. A hint to the route from becoming to being is in the words themselves.* Come *means to travel toward a target. By eliminating the effort to travel toward something different and embracing and being grateful for what is, the striving in* becoming *disappears and you are left with* being.[8]

The three Being practices will help you wake up and integrate present-moment awareness into your everyday life.

The Origins of Being

Henry David Thoreau's two-year, two-month "sojourn" at Walden Pond was one of the great experiments in being. Thoreau was inspired to escape to Walden because he felt his fellow townspeople lived in a sleeping state. He viewed them as "overcome with drowsiness" and distracted by "petty fears and petty pleasures." This ordinary state of distraction came at a high cost: "Our life," said Thoreau, "is frittered away by detail."[9] We miss out on the beauty of each moment, he thought, not because we have something better to do, but because we're preoccupied with the "shams and delusions" of the mind.

These perceptions led Thoreau to leave society in hopes of learning how to wake up. "I went to the woods because I wished to live deliberately, to front only the essential facts of life, and see if I could not learn what it had to teach, and not, when I came to die, discover that I had not lived." His goal was to "live deep and suck out all the marrow of life."[10]

Thoreau did many things during his time at Walden. He writes in excruciating detail about hoeing beans, sweeping the floor, and other mundane tasks like surveying the depth of the pond. To focus on what he did, however, would be to miss the point. The book isn't really about what he did but *how* he did it. It's about what life looks like when each moment becomes an opportunity to wake up and be fully here. It's a book about being.

You don't need to leave your family and your job and move to the woods to get a taste of this experience. Every day is filled with thousands of opportunities to experience this moment: while taking a shower, brushing your teeth, or driving to work. Thoreau's challenge is to realize that our wellbeing has less to do with what we are doing and more to do with *how* we do it. If we learn to wake up in the midst of our ordinary life, sitting in traffic, waiting in a long line, and other everyday moments can become opportunities to shift our experience of being. Thoreau's lesson to us is that waking up requires us to look inside ourselves to experience the fullness of wellbeing. It is not dependent on the external circumstances and conditions of our lives.

Of course, this idea of waking up to being isn't unique to Thoreau. Most spiritual and philosophical traditions describe similar divisions between ordinary and divine, sacred and profane, sleeping and waking, the screen and the projection. Thoreau himself found inspiration in the spiritual traditions of the East, which use the very same metaphor of waking up. In fact, the word *Buddha* means "awakened one."

Hindu texts point to a similar idea. They portray us as slumbering in the realm of *maya,* "illusion" or "not that." The Bhagavad Gita says that God's "maya makes all beings revolve as if on a potter's machine,"[11] spinning endlessly through our lives. To shift out of maya is to begin to wake up.

Ancient Western thinkers also pointed to this key shift in being. In the *Apology,* Socrates said that his technique of questioning was aimed at waking up the citizens of Athens: "I awaken and persuade and reproach each one of you, and I do not stop settling down everywhere upon you the whole day." Without him, he told the people of Athens, "you would spend the rest of your lives asleep."[12]

We have all experienced the difference between the sleeping and waking state of being that the ancients describe. To begin spending more time feeling awake to each moment, you will learn three practices designed to help you shift into being by developing the skill of attention. These Be Stage practices will help you catch yourself when your mind wanders and bring your focus back to the present moment. The next chapter will introduce you to a core inner technology of LIFE XT that will help you make this shift anytime, anywhere—a tool we call Notice-Shift-Rewire.

NOTICE-SHIFT-REWIRE

Alan and Gina sit on the beach, gazing out over the sparkling blue sea before them. But that's pretty much the only thing they have in common.

Alan feels grateful just to be able to spend these few precious hours soaking in the view, listening to the soft crash of each wave and the squawking of gulls overhead, feeling the warmth of the rough sand on his legs and the sensation of the breeze against his skin. He spends a few minutes contemplating the things he needs to do when he gets home—the quick trip to the grocery store, the call to his sister, and some necessary yard work—but these thoughts dissipate as he brings himself back to the sea, the waves, the sand, and the breeze, feeling relaxed and connected to the present moment.

Gina looks out at the very same ocean, listening to music through her earbuds while alternating between playing an addictive game on her phone and skimming the latest action on her Facebook and Twitter pages. Gina is happy to be out in the sun, happy to have some downtime, but each time she puts down her phone, thoughts flood into her mind. She thinks about how she'd like to change jobs, worries about what her boyfriend is doing, and wonders when she will have more time to relax. For a second or two, her thoughts cease and she looks in amazement at the crease of the horizon, where sky meets sea. *It's so beautiful.* But then—*wham!*—

she's thinking about the last time she was here, with Tim, and they had that argument that led to a breakup, which meant she had to move into that less-than-optimal apartment she's in now, which really needs some paint . . . And just like that, she's no longer at the beach; she's time-traveling through her mind.

Living Life Cross Training

Most of us swing back and forth between Alan's exquisite experience of the present moment and Gina's scattered and distracted state of mind. In one moment we feel relaxed and connected to what we're doing now; in the next we're distracted by a friend's harsh comment in an email yesterday or we're already worrying about the meeting we have to attend in half an hour.

In the Train Stage, we introduced essential tools for navigating these waves of the mind. Meditation trains the skill of focused attention. Movement enhances the neurobiological background of our experience or, as Thoreau phrased it, "puts sunshine into our thoughts." Inquiry helps loosen the hold of the stressful thoughts that arise.

But mastering the Train Stage practices isn't the ultimate goal. LIFE XT isn't about becoming a master meditator or an accomplished athlete, though that might happen along the way. Our goal is much more profound: It is to live each day—indeed, each moment—with a greater sense of wellbeing.

Attaining this larger goal requires complementing the Train Stage practices with a different kind of practice. It requires developing the moment-to-moment habit of attention—a habit you will master using the inner technology of Notice-Shift-Rewire. This one skill sits at the core of all of LIFE XT.

- *Noticing* our mental habits brings choice. We can now choose where to place our attention.
- *Shifting* brings change.
- *Rewiring* brings lasting neurological integration.

Together, this inner technology allows us to release the forces of the set point by shaping our experience of each moment.

Mind Wandering

What keeps us from living this moment-to-moment experience of being and doing? The short answer: mind wandering. If our minds were perpetually still and always focused on the object of our choosing, we could easily experience the fullness of each moment and stay focused on giving our greatest contribution. Being and doing would be easy.

For most of us, however, that isn't the case. We experience what Buddhists call the *monkey mind*. Elizabeth Gilbert, author of the bestselling memoir *Eat, Pray, Love*, talks about her experience of this scattered state of mind:

> *I am burdened with . . . the monkey mind. The thoughts that swing from limb to limb, stopping only to scratch themselves, spit and howl. My mind swings wildly through time, touching on dozens of ideas a minute, unharnessed and undisciplined.*[1]

Byron Katie describes this by saying, "We aren't thinking. We are being thought."[2] To greater or lesser degrees, all of us experience this universal human condition. Modern psychologists call this mind wandering. It's what happens when our attention runs on autopilot, drifting from random musings about our past to anxiety-producing what-ifs about the future. In this state, we live with the constant distraction of that crazy, unrelenting inner voice that keeps the mind in a perpetual state of wandering.

Of course, not all mind wandering is bad. Research shows that allowing your mind to dwell on creative problems or important future events can have positive benefits.[3] Allowing your mind to explore a problem you are facing at work can lead to important and unexpected insights. Allowing your mind to explore possible itineraries for an upcoming vacation can ensure smooth travels. These more focused forms of thinking correspond to what many ancient traditions call contemplation. In these states, the mind may wander, but it doesn't run wild.

In the course of everyday life, however, we tend to experience a different, more problematic form of mind wandering. Our mind isn't contemplating profound intellectual breakthroughs or important future priorities. It's ruminating aimlessly through mostly negative terrain. This near-constant stream of everyday mind wandering diminishes our emotional wellbeing.

A Harvard University study conducted in 2010 by Matthew A. Killingsworth and Daniel T. Gilbert revealed that most of us mind wander—a lot. In fact, the average person spends 47 percent of the day mind wandering: thinking about something other than his or her present activity. The bulk of this mind wandering is focused on pleasant thoughts (42.5 percent), while the rest is divided between neutral thoughts (31 percent) and unpleasant thoughts (26.5 percent).[5]

Their key insight wasn't just that our minds wander. It was the link between mind wandering and unhappiness. Killingsworth concluded, "How often our minds leave the present and where they tend to go is a better predictor of our happiness than the activities in which we are engaged."[6] Mind wandering doesn't just stand in the way of enjoying an ocean-front view. This landmark study shows that it stands in the way of happiness.[7]

The Modern Dilemma

Mind wandering is an ancient human problem. But today's high-tech environment, far from giving us more free time, is actually reinforcing our mind's tendency to wander. Distractions like email, texting, social networking, video games, movies, and the rapid pace of life offer a constant invitation to inattention.

The Inner Technology of Notice-Shift-Rewire

The first three practices of the Train Stage—Meditation, Movement, and Inquiry—require that you set aside time. You can't meditate in the middle of an important client meeting. You can't exercise in a crowded airplane. To do these practices, you need to take a short break from the activities of ordinary life. And as you now know, the time and effort is worth it: These practices are essential to training the skill of wellbeing.

By contrast, Notice-Shift-Rewire is a tool of life integration—a tool designed to be used anytime, anywhere. It's meant to help you shift back to the state of being and doing while you are in the midst of your day-to-day life. Think of it as meditation in motion. Like sitting meditation, it trains the skill of attention. Unlike meditation, it can be done anytime, anywhere. In every moment, after all, your attention is directed somewhere. When you're walking down the stairs, combing your hair, even right now, as you are reading this sentence, your mind is either wandering or focused. When the mind wanders, Notice-Shift-Rewire is the tool that brings us back.

The practice is straightforward.

- *Notice* when the mind wanders.
- *Shift* the mind back to your chosen object of concentration.
- *Rewire* the brain's neural pathways by savoring this new experience.

Notice-Shift-Rewire is the most fundamental skill that you will train in all of LIFE XT—a skill that you can draw on in just about any situation: while shopping at the grocery store, shoveling snow, or getting crammed into the back corner of a crowded elevator. When we learn the art of Notice-Shift-Rewire, we learn to become the conductors of our own attention, shifting from mind wandering to the six states of being and doing. Here's how it works:

Step 1: Notice

It all starts with Noticing. Noticing is the act of observing the mind—of standing back and watching the set point forces at work. The spiritual traditions use words like *witnessing, consciousness,* and *awareness* to describe this state of mind.

This is not the usual human state. The forces of the set point can leave us lost in the stories our minds tell us, trapped in judgment, attachment, and resistance. When these habitual patterns of thought govern our behavior, it's difficult to improve our general sense of wellbeing.

Noticing—simple, nonjudgmental awareness—is key to establishing a new habit of being. It allows us to put the critic aside and discover a less used part of our consciousness: the neutral watcher. The watcher is able to take a step back and see what is happening in the mind. This act of awareness—of watching what is going on in the mind—is the first step to training the skill of attention. It opens the possibility for the next step: shifting.

Step 2: Shift

Shifting—redirecting your attention—is the action that creates the change. Suppose you just had a long, difficult day at work. You feel discouraged, exhausted. Marching through your consciousness is an army of judgments: *I am so tired. I wish I had a different job. If only I had more time.* These thoughts do nothing but drain your energy. Simply noticing—*I feel discouraged; I feel tired; it was a long day*—is where you start.

Once you have noticed, you have a choice. You can let these habits of the set point run the show, or you can choose to shift. You might shift your attention to any one of the Being and Doing practices we describe later in *Start Here.* You can shift to Gratitude by savoring the feeling of appreciation for your family, your home, or your good health. Alternatively, you might shift to Presence by focusing on the sensation of your breath or the sound of the wind rustling the trees. Shifting enables you to redirect your attention— from the wanderings of the mind to qualities that promote well-being.

The word *shift* might make you think that the goal here is to shift *away* from what's happening right now. This is a common misconception. The goal here isn't to repress or check out of your current experience. The goal is to check *in*—to draw your attention away from the haphazard musings of the mind and into what is actually happening right now. When we shift, we meet what is with complete equanimity.

Step 3: Rewire

Now we come to the part where the long-term payoffs reside. In Step 3, we begin to rewire the brain's neural pathways by taking a brief moment to savor the new experience that arises after making a shift. By spending just fifteen to thirty seconds savoring the shift, you keep these productive neural pathways firing and help encode a heightened experience of wellbeing deep into your brain and nervous system. You set in motion the process of neural integration—of creating new, more powerful pathways of activation in the brain.[8]

The Challenge of Notice-Shift-Rewire

Notice-Shift-Rewire is a skill that sounds easy. But it requires practice to develop. When we first started developing and experimenting with the practice, we both fell into the trap of thinking that we could spend every waking moment applying this skill. The results were disastrous: We found that we could barely make it an hour, let alone five minutes, without slipping back into mind wandering. As Nate explains:

> When I started training Notice-Shift-Rewire, I really thought I could train myself to do it all the time—to be present, grateful, and compassionate in every moment. It didn't work out that way—not even close. I might remember to Notice-Shift-Rewire at various points throughout the day. But then, minutes later, I would get lost in a sea of thoughts. Trying to do this all the time—in every situation—turned out to be a recipe for failure. The breakthrough occurred when Eric and I began researching the science of habit formation

and realized that using a few everyday cues would be a better way to form this habit. So instead of trying to Notice-Shift-Rewire all day, we adopted the more reasonable goal of doing it in response to a cue: while showering, eating, or leaving the house. This changed everything. After a few weeks, I had created a habit in these situations, and eventually I started to remember to Notice-Shift-Rewire more often in the rest of my life.

We learned from these early experiments that it is more realistic and helpful to develop specific habits of Notice-Shift-Rewire. In the following chapters, you will use specific habit-forming cues to apply Notice-Shift-Rewire not only to the three Being practices but also to further reinforce the three Doing practices. By the end of the program, this skill will become second nature.

The Science of Notice-Shift-Rewire

"Neurons that fire together, wire together"

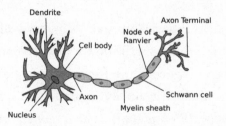

Your brain is made up of around 100 billion neurons. These tiny cells work as the messengers of the brain, relaying electrochemical messages through the synapses to other neurons. When a neuron receives enough excitation, it generates an electrical and chemical pulse that moves through the axon and in turn activates the synapses of other neurons. Viewing this mechanism as a simple on-off switch helps illustrate how change can begin to occur.

(continued on next page)

Donald Hebb, one of the pioneers in the field, explains: "When an axon of cell A is near enough to excite a cell B and repeatedly or persistently takes part in firing it, some growth process or metabolic change takes place in one or both cells such that A's efficiency, as one of the cells firing B, is increased."[9] Put simply, "neurons that fire together wire together."

By activating a new network of neurons repeatedly, we create metabolic changes in the brain and grow new networks of activation. This is the core principle behind Notice-Shift-Rewire. At the beginning, your capacity for attention may be inefficient and difficult to access. But when practiced consistently, this inner technology becomes a tool to help us improve the skill of attention and, in so doing, creates new networks of activation that grow in strength and efficiency over time. Dan Siegel, one of the foremost researchers on the neuroscience of mindfulness, observes, "When we focus our attention in specific ways, we create neural firing patterns that permit previously separated areas to become linked and integrated."[10]

The Wisdom and Science of Notice-Shift-Rewire

For thousands of years, wisdom traditions have offered a remarkably similar set of insights on the power of attention—the core skill that we train using Notice-Shift-Rewire. Throughout these works, a similar theme emerges again and again: *When we allow the mind to wander, we suffer. When we learn to direct our attention, we improve our wellbeing.*

In the Dhammapada, the Buddha likens the power of the elephant to the power of the mind. The mind is also capable of amazing things. But without discipline and training, it roams all over the place, like an untrained animal. "Long ago," the Buddha declares, "my mind used to wander as it liked and do what it wanted. Now I can rule my mind as the mahout controls the elephant with his hooked staff." [11] While you won't find references to Notice-Shift-Rewire in these ancient texts, the Buddha's reflections point to a similar way of training the mind. "Be vigilant," he insists, "guard your mind against negative thoughts. Pull yourself out of bad ways as an elephant raises itself out of the mud." [12]

Aristotle expressed a similar enthusiasm for the power of attention. At the beginning of *The Nicomachean Ethics*, he asked, "Are we not more likely to achieve our aim if we have a target? Every art and every investigation, and similarly every action and pursuit, is considered to aim at some good." [13] Here Aristotle makes the case that it is the capacity of attention that allows us to hit the target.

Long before there were fMRI machines, the American poet and philosopher Ralph Waldo Emerson brilliantly foreshadowed the neurobiological benefits of developing this skill of attention. "When a strong will appears," says Emerson, "it usually results from a certain unity of organization, as if the whole energy of body and mind flowed in one direction." [14] Ancient wisdom is clear: the antidote to mind wandering is to learn to develop this "unity of organization" and direct our attention.

The skill that we call attention corresponds to what neuroscientists call *executive attention*, a capacity that enables us to sort through conflicting stimuli. If you are walking through Times Square in New York City, for example, executive attention is the faculty of the mind that allows your brain to remain focused on your destination rather than the car horns, billboards, and bright lights that surround you.

When executive attention is weak, we become more impulsive, rigid, and susceptible to worry, fear, and other symptoms of psychological distress. Our minds easily lose the capacity to resolve conflicts among competing stimuli, leaving us distracted, scattered, and tense.

The good news is that modern science now shows that we can learn the skill of developing executive attention throughout life. When we train the skill of attention, we actually change our brains by activating new neural connections that reduce mind wandering and enhance overall wellbeing.

Training the quality of attention is a lot like training a muscle: The more we train it, the stronger it becomes. Each time we Notice-Shift-Rewire from mind wandering to attention we strengthen this capacity.[15] Think of NSR as doing push-ups for your brain.

PRACTICE 4: PRESENCE

In the late 1980s, South African music journalist Michael Brown lived what he called a "blissfully unconscious life." Then one day, while he was driving to a venue, everything changed. It started with a sharp, throbbing pain in his eye. Within minutes, the pain became so excruciating that he had to stop the car and throw up on the side of the road.

When the pain subsided, Brown wrote it off as a freak event. But then it came back again and again and again. Brown searched out the top doctors and neurologists in South Africa. After two years, he was diagnosed with a rare neurological condition called Horton's syndrome, a condition for which there is no known cause and no known cure.

Brown's prognosis looked bleak. For the next ten years, Brown searched for a cure for this painful condition. He used a variety of prescription medications, removed his wisdom teeth, and even received cortisone injections in his face. Nothing worked. He still lived in intense pain.

Then one day Brown had a life-changing insight: He learned that when he was truly present—awake to the experience of this moment—the pain started to dissolve. When he was distracted or out of the moment, the pain intensified.

This insight led Brown to devote his life to training the skill of presence, using each situation as an opportunity to get present. By learning to become "increasingly present," says Brown, "the intensity of my painful condition continued to subside. After years of suffering from this neurological agony—and the frustration, anxiety, anger, grief, and depression it seeded—a light was now shining in the darkness."[1]

Today Brown no longer experiences the painful symptoms of Horton's syndrome. He cured his chronic condition by training a profound skill—by learning to use each moment as an opportunity to shift from the wandering mind to the experience of presence, of what is here and now.

Brown's story seems almost magical, but it is well within our reach. In fact, ancient wisdom traditions have documented such experiences for thousands of years. More recently, modern science has begun to validate this age-old practice, and millions of people have benefited from presence-based practices like mindfulness-based stress reduction (MBSR) and dialectical behavior therapy (DBT).

The key insight is this: When we take the stillness from our meditation practice into our everyday lives and shift from the busyness of the mind to this moment, a powerful and almost magical change occurs. We begin to see our lives with greater clarity and to experience more ease, confidence, and wellbeing, while also becoming more focused, productive, and attentive. Through developing the habit of presence, we get in touch with the fundamental wonder of what it is to be alive, and even the most ordinary moments become extraordinary. The Presence practice will help you train this life-enhancing skill.

WHAT IT IS

Presence is meditation in motion, meditation in the midst of day-to-day life.

When meditating, we typically become still. We remove ourselves from the chaos of everyday life: no emails, no calls, no kids, no distractions.

Presence is the practice of bringing this meditative mindfulness into the activities of everyday life. We can practice this art of being here now while waiting in a long grocery store checkout line, changing a baby's diaper, or sitting in bumper-to-bumper traffic.

Presence involves a simple yet incredible shift—from the ordinary state of mind wandering to bringing our attention to the experience of what is happening right now. You can make this shift anytime, anywhere. In fact you can try it right now. When you finish reading this paragraph, put down the book for thirty seconds. Simply pay attention to what's happening in this moment. Notice your breath. Notice the sounds. Notice the sensations in your body.

Now notice how you feel. That's the experience of presence.

Why develop this habit? Spiritual teachers and philosophers have attempted to answer this question for thousands of years. And yet Ferris Bueller—the impetuous high school student from the classic 1986 film—might just have the best answer: "Life moves pretty fast," he warned. "If you don't stop and look around for a while, you might miss it."

He's right. Life without presence moves pretty fast. When we wake up, go to work, and do the other things we need to do, we often operate on autopilot; the days fly by, as do the weeks, months, and years. In fact, scientists have confirmed that this experience of time "flying by" increases with age. With each passing year, the novelty of life diminishes and our perception of time accelerates.[2]

This has led the mindfulness teacher Jon Kabat-Zinn to argue that if you really want to live a longer life, presence—not drugs, healthy eating, or any other strategy—is the best solution. You may not actually live longer in terms of calendar time, but your experience of life and your perception of time will expand. The days, months, and years will be richer, more meaningful, more fully lived.

Appreciating the fall leaves, listening to the crunch of your feet as you walk on the winter snow, smelling the scents of the early spring air, and feeling the warmth of the summer sun—these simple acts of presence slow life down. They help us go through each day feeling more alive, awake, and content.

There are other benefits, too. Presence doesn't simply change the quality of being. As you will see in the Engagement practice, it can also transform the quality of doing. It leads to increased productivity, greater creative flow, and enhanced relationships.

Although Presence is a practice with profound benefits, it isn't always easy to make this shift. As we practice Presence, we must navigate not only mental distractions (as in meditation) but also the many distractions of the outside world: cell phones, car horns, and airport delays.

Meredith, a mother of two young boys and marketing strategist, tells us about the challenges she faces in practicing Presence:

Despite having spent most of the last decade exploring various forms of spiritual practice, my grasp on the present moment is still tenuous. I'd like to classify myself as a "seeker," but mostly I'm an entrepreneur and a busy mom. My time is filled with tasks and to-do lists and my mind is often filled with those sneaky, meandering thoughts about my crow's-feet, the extra five pounds in the middle, and what to wear to XYZ event. I often laugh and say that I could have earned a Nobel Prize with all the time I've wasted thinking about clothes. Sometimes, though, in the midst of work, rushing to pick up my son, and random musings about fashion, as if out of nowhere, I have brief moments where everything slows down. I feel grateful for my kids, connected to them, and happy to be here. For a moment, the chaos stops. Until it starts up again . . .

Like most of us, Meredith lives a hectic life. And yet these occasional moments of presence allow her to slow down the hands of time—to feel connection, gratitude, and joy.

The Presence practice is based on the idea that we can train ourselves to experience more of the kind of moments Meredith describes. The practice uses the inner technology of Notice-Shift-Rewire to redirect our attention in the midst of day-to-day life: as you pull out of the driveway, button a shirt, or wait to use a cash machine at the bank. To help build the habit and remember to do it each day, you will work with an ordinary life cue: taking a shower or bathing. Each day you will use showering as your prompt for shifting your attention to the sights, sounds, and sensations happening right now.

WHY IT WORKS

Many clichés surround the idea of presence. Live in the moment, be mindful, carpe diem, and the social-media-inspired YOLO (you only live once). These slogans, which appear in everything from greeting cards to hip-hop lyrics, can make this state of mind sound flaky and unproductive, something that happens only while you are lying on the beach or sitting alone in the woods in a state of complete inactivity.

So what is the present moment? This almost sounds like a trick question. Everyone knows that the present moment is what is happening now. It's the wind in the trees, the touch of fabric against your skin, the hummingbird feeding by your window.

But it's not that simple. There's also something quite mysterious about this moment. It's not like the past, which stretches infinitely behind us. It's also not like the future, which stretches infinitely ahead. In fact, the moment you try to capture it, it's gone. It becomes just another part of the past.

This quandary led the American philosopher John Dewey to question whether the present moment even exists: "Each moment of experience confesses itself to be a transition between two worlds, the immediate past and the immediate future."[3] What we call the present moment, he observed, is an ephemeral, almost nonexistent instant that is swallowed up by what comes before and after it.

Like Dewey, many ancient Stoic philosophers saw the present as infinitely thin—so fine that it almost ceases to exist.[4] But unlike Dewey, they saw it as also having infinite depth. Pierre Hadot, one of the most influential living scholars of ancient thought, observes that for the ancient Stoic philosophers, "The present represented a certain 'thickness' of time,"[5] even as it sits on the knife-edge between past and future. If we can train ourselves to draw all of our attention to this delicate slice of time, the Stoics observed, we can radically shift our mental state—we can experience sublime well-being.

In fact, the ancient Greeks identified three ways that opening to the present moment increases the depth of our experience and productive possibilities of each moment. First, when we fully experience what is here and now, we no longer postpone what we most want. We live our fullest life *now*. The philosopher Epicurus captures this ethos of urgency:

> *We are only born once—twice is not allowed—and it is necessary that we shall be no more, for all eternity; and yet you, who are not master of tomorrow, you keep on putting off your joy?*[6]

This is something that many of us have experienced. Have you ever heard the shocking and sad news that someone close to you died and then thought, *Am I living my life as fully and as presently possible?* Death makes us acutely aware of our aliveness and the preciousness of each moment.

Second, attending to the present moment enables us to take advantage of the full range of possibilities that exist in each moment. The Greeks used the word *kairos* to describe the power in each moment.[7] If we're stuck in past or future, the possibilities open to us in this moment disappear. If we enter the present, however, we can spontaneously adapt to even the most challenging situations. If you're stuck at the airport, waiting out a three-hour flight delay, for example, you can let the mind swirl with thoughts about past and future: *I should have taken the earlier flight* or *I'm going to be so late.* Or you can experience *kairos.* You can take advantage of the new possibilities available to you as a result of the three-hour delay: power walking through the concourse, reading for pleasure, or catching up with old friends on the phone.

Getting present also opens up a third possibility: *happiness and wellbeing,* the destination of LIFE XT. When we spend the day traveling through past and future, we tend to get trapped in a host of negative emotions, from anxiety to irritation to resentment. The Epicurean school of ancient Greek thought used sayings like the following to illustrate this point: "Senseless people live in hope for the future, and since this cannot be certain, they are consumed by fear and anxiety"[8]

When we manage to enter the razor-thin moment of presence, something amazing happens: these anxieties and resentments dissolve. We experience ease, equanimity, and peace. In short, we experience wellbeing. As Marcus Aurelius declared, "All the happiness you are trying to achieve by long, roundabout ways: you can have it all right now . . . that is, if you leave everything past behind you, entrust the future to providence, and if you arrange the present in accordance with piety and justice."[9]

When we enter fully into the present moment, something incredible happens. Our regrets and anxieties begin to melt, and we experience a greater sense of aliveness, an enhanced capacity to take full advantage of the possibilities of each moment, and above all, profound wellbeing.

HOW TO DEVELOP THIS SKILL

Habit 4: Presence

How to do it: All of the LIFE XT practices, including the practice of Presence, are derived from the science of habit formation (for more see Appendix 1). Like each of the Being practices, Presence involves using a cue from everyday life as the trigger to Notice-Shift-Rewire your attention. For the practice of Presence, use showering as your cue to Notice-Shift-Rewire to the present moment. Notice—see if you can become aware—each time you step into the shower. Shift

(continued on next page)

your attention to the sights, sounds, and sensations of the present moment. Feel the warmth of the water, hear the sound it makes as it falls from the shower head to the hard ground below. Rewire by savoring this experience.

Why showering? you might be asking yourself. A few reasons. First, showering is something that most of us do every day. Second, the shower is one of the last refuges from the distractions of modern life: smartphones, tablets, TVs, and the Internet. Finally, showering takes time—around eight minutes for the average American. This gives you an extended opportunity to experience presence. In fact, you can use your daily shower as a kind of mini-meditation on presence that fits easily and efficiently into your daily routine. If showering isn't the right cue for you, feel free to pick some other daily activity. Just be sure to be consistent: Use the same cue each day to form the habit of Presence.

For more tips and strategies for building this habit, see the discussion of Presence in the chapter "How To Practice Life Cross Training" at the end of the book.

Out of the Shower: Presence in the Rest of Life

Remember, presence is something you can experience anytime, anywhere. It's not a distraction or a way of checking out from the activities of everyday life. Instead, it's a way of checking in and experiencing these activities more fully. It's the inner equivalent of focusing a camera on a previously blurry image or upgrading from standard cable to HD. The sights, sounds, and sensations of reality stay the same. The shift to presence simply makes them come to life with a deep vibrancy and profound awareness.

To access this shift in just about any situation, use the inner technology of Notice-Shift-Rewire.

Step 1: Notice

Noticing is the magical moment of being. When we notice, we immediately become aware of our thoughts and become present. This awareness opens the possibility for a shift out of the set point mind and into a more sustained state of presence. You can start with just one second of presence. With practice, these periods will become longer and longer.

Throughout the day, try to catch yourself when you get lost in the tangled loops of past and future. As you will soon see, this happens thousands of times each day, and most of the time we are completely unaware that it is even happening. So don't worry about catching yourself every time your mind wanders. Start by training the habit of presence in the shower, then see if you can catch yourself a few more times throughout the day.

Step 2: Shift

Once you notice your mind wandering, a shift has naturally occurred. The next step is to deepen this shift and expand the moment. There is no single portal into the present moment. In fact, you can use anything that's happening right now (as opposed to the time-traveling ruminations of the mind) as your way in. Here are some of the possibilities:

- *Breath.* As with meditation, the breath can be a useful tool. The breath is your anchor back to this moment. It's the part of you that is always happening right now.
- *Sounds.* Focus on the sounds happening right now: on the clock ticking in the background, the tapping of keys on your computer keyboard, or the sound of the wind rustling the leaves.

- *Sights.* Focus on the sights happening right now: on the color of the walls, the shape of the clouds, the texture of the ground.
- *Bodily sensations.* Focus on the sensations in the body: on the tingles, twinges, and tight spots in the body, or the feeling of your feet on the floor.

Margi, a retired IT specialist, offers insight into how the sense of touch helps her be in the present moment:

Gardening has been a source of joy and creativity for years. Designing the garden, providing the proper food and water, weeding, and working with the plants allows me to be more present and at ease. I feel the cool sensation of the dirt against my skin. I feel the texture of the leaves of each plant. I feel the dampness of freshly watered soil. I no longer worry about what I need to do later that day. I'm just there—in the garden, feeling the sensations of earth.

Margi's story offers a reminder that it doesn't matter what you attend to. The key is to identify your own set of moves away from mental time-traveling and into this moment.

Step 3: Rewire

Once you notice and shift your attention to deepen your awareness and experience of this moment, take a brief instant to savor this shift and experience the poetry of the moment—its unique qualities. Spend thirty seconds enjoying the feeling of your breath moving in and out. Spend a minute taking in the sights around you.

The Advanced Practice

It is difficult to stay present in the midst of your everyday life—while you rush out the door or stand in a long airport security line. But this training will also help you cultivate an even more challenging skill—staying present in the midst of intense emotions like anger, sadness, or fear.

This practice runs counter to many of our most deeply ingrained coping habits. When we feel intense emotion, we tend to do just about anything we can to avoid experiencing it fully. We watch TV, check our phone, go on Facebook, have a drink, or even use practices like movement to get rid of the discomfort.

There is, however, enormous benefit in learning to be present in these states. If we push them away, we empower them. Our attachment to "good" states of positive emotion increases along with our resistance to "bad" states of negative emotion. If we learn to be present with the sensations that arise in the midst of fear, sadness, anger, and other uncomfortable states, we can learn to become more open to these experiences. We learn that they are simply "e-motions"—life energy in motion.[10] We learn that these states can be a gateway to deeper insight and a richer engagement in life.

So the advanced presence practice is to train to become and remain present in the midst of these most challenging states. It is "advanced" because the terrain of these states is much rougher and trickier to navigate than ordinary states. The human habit is to feel the discomfort of fear or sadness and then try to make sense of it by getting lost in a mind-generated loop of thoughts—a mental echo that rings on and on for hours. To get present with these states is to drop the stories and directly experience the uncomfortable feelings and sensations that go along with fear, shame, longing, sadness, or anger.

Pema Chödrön, the prolific author and teacher, offers some helpful advice:

Most of us will find that we can only do it in small bites because the shaky, tender feeling can be so intense and so gut wrenching and so unnerving. The gentle approach is to just take it in small bites. Spend just a few seconds standing in your own shoes fully when your knees are shaking and you can hardly speak; just stay present with that feeling of fear or terror for even a few seconds. Each time you are daring in this way . . . it opens up new neurological pathways in the brain. You experience that as strength, as easier to do it the next time.[11]

Take it slow. See if you can stay present in the midst of these intense emotions for just a few moments. The key move is to learn to distinguish between sensation and story. The felt sensation of emotion in the body happens in the present moment. The stories that arise in the mind, by contrast, pull us out of present time. The key to this practice is to notice the stories your mind generates. You can even label them as *stories* or *thinking*. Then shift your attention back to the sensations in the body. Watch the internal experience of emotion. Locate it in your body. Just a second of this kind of presence will change your habitual way of reacting and make it easier to stay present the next time.

With time, you will gain confidence in your ability to apply Notice-Shift-Rewire to presence in the midst of even the most uncomfortable, scary, or challenging experiences. And it is this confidence that lays the groundwork for living a life of fearlessness. Chödrön explains, "The only way to experience fearlessness is to know the nature of fear. Fear is not something we get rid of or cast out. It is something we can come to know so well that the journey of knowing fear, moving closer to fear, is in fact the basis of fear-lessness."[12]

Imagine for a moment what your life will be like when you learn how to stay present and drop your resistance to fear, sadness, shame, and anger. Imagine letting these states come and go, like waves in the ocean. This is a deep state of contentment that you can begin to experience through the advanced practice.

WHAT TO EXPECT

As you develop the habit of Notice-Shift-Rewire, you will slowly develop the habit of presence both when you take a shower and in the rest of your life.

We have found that a couple of distinct stages arise on the journey of developing presence. The first is the stage of habit formation. This stage lasts anywhere from a couple of weeks to a month. At the very beginning of this stage, your experience of presence may feel forced and unnatural. You will need to expend some real willpower to remember to do it each day and remember to track your progress. After a few weeks, however, the efficiency-boosting benefits of habit will start to kick in. You don't need to work quite so hard to remember. In fact, when you step into your shower, you start to experience presence without really even thinking about it.

The next stage is stabilization. Once the habit is formed, it's essential to continue doing it every day. Like any new habit, if you stop, you will lose the momentum you have built during the initial stage. If you keep it up, you can expect to begin experiencing spontaneous moments of presence throughout the day. Every micro-moment of presence, after all, has a profound effect. Using Notice-Shift-Rewire to redirect your attention to presence as you shower each day will soon lead to using it ten times each day in other everyday life situations. Using it ten times each day leads to a new mental habit of shifting to presence hundreds of times each day, even if only for an instant. This is the way wellbeing arises—as the Buddha famously described it, drop by drop, moment by moment.[13] A single second of presence is like a single drop filling a water pot. It may not fill the pot right away—but it matters. Over time, as the drops become more frequent, as presence becomes a habit, the pot will fill: You will experience less stress, worry, and other symptoms of the wandering mind and more of the sounds, sights, smells, and sensations happening right now.

The result will be more unplanned and unexpected moments of being here now. Adam, a tech intern and advanced LIFE XT practitioner, shares his experience of one such spontaneous moment of presence:

I had locked myself in my apartment for a couple of days, trying to finish a tech development application in time for a presentation the next day. It was coming down to the eleventh hour, and it felt like every bug I fixed created two more in the process. I was beyond frustrated and desperately needed to clear my mind. I threw on a light jacket and left the apartment, stepping out into the damp and dreary night. The rain had subsided to a light drizzle with an occasional rumble of thunder. I could sense the encroaching cloudiness of my thoughts as my mind aimlessly continued to debug as I walked. Then in an instant, I "woke up" to the world around me. All worried thoughts and expectations fell away to the simplicity of Now. I was absorbed in the moment, feeling each raindrop as it struck my skin. The air I breathed felt fresher as it filled my lungs. I could focus my entire attention on the speckled white noise created by thousands of drops hitting the earth at once. It was awesome. When I returned to my apartment, I was more focused and was able to quickly complete my task.

Adam's story points to an experience that will become increasingly familiar to you as you develop and stabilize this habit. It also points to the primary challenge that you may encounter along the way: the challenge of attachment.

Presence is an amazing experience. The more you taste it, the more you may want to feast on it. We encountered this attachment to presence early on and it led us to believe that we could experience this state all the time—that we could somehow replace ordinary mind wandering with presence. We have learned that this is a recipe for failure. It's the same as thinking that you can get rid of all your thoughts by meditating. It's impossible.

The antidote to this challenge is to accept the paradox of presence. Enjoy the moments of presence that do arise, but accept the fact that you will still get distracted and caught in the loops of the mind—that you can't be in the moment all the time. Don't try to hold on to this exquisite experience. Just enjoy these moments when they do arise and allow them to come and go.

PRACTICE 5: GRATITUDE

Stephen King has much to be grateful for. He is one of the most widely read horror and suspense writers of all time and has achieved international acclaim for his many books and the movies based on them. But above all else, Stephen King is grateful simply to be alive.

In June 1999, King was strolling along one of the country roads near his lake house in western Maine. A little farther up the road, the driver of a blue minivan took his eyes off the road to keep his dog from getting into his cooler. As King looked up, the minivan was bearing down on him so fast he had no time to jump out of the way. He bounced off the windshield, landing on the ground in a blur.[1]

King lay on the side of the road as blood gushed from his head. A bone in his right leg protruded out of his jeans. The driver told King that he had never received so much as a parking ticket (a claim later revealed to be false). King responded, "Well, I've never been hit by a car before."[2]

The accident left King with a fractured hip, a scalp laceration, multiple fractures in his right leg, and four broken ribs. At first the doctors weren't sure if he would ever walk again; they even contemplated amputating his leg.

King's condition gave him every excuse to dwell on the negative. No one would have blamed him for wallowing in thoughts like *The driver of that minivan did this to me*, *It's not fair*, or *This shouldn't have happened.* But for King, this accident had a very different out-come. It didn't leave him with bitterness or resentment. Just one year after the accident, he remarked:

> *I'm grateful for everything that I have, and I try to stay as grateful as I can, because it doesn't matter how much money you've made or how rich you are or whether your book's on the Internet or anything else. If you snap your spine, you're a quadriplegic, and mine was chipped in five or six places, almost down to the bare wires in a couple of places. So I'm very lucky.*[3]

In spite of the pain, the scars, and the long road to healing, King experienced something profound as a result of what happened on that June day in 1999: the happiness-inducing power of gratitude.

Gateway to Gratitude

Let's see if you can experience this feeling yourself, right here, right now.

Take a moment to write down three things on a sheet of paper that you find irritating or annoying in this moment. It might be the background hum of an air-conditioning unit, a subtle feeling of discomfort in your stomach, or the lingering sting of your coworker's comment at yesterday's meeting.

1. _____

2. _____

3. _____

Now take fifteen to thirty seconds to focus on these three irritants, one by one. Pay close attention to any associated emotions or sensations.

Now check in. How do you feel? Do you feel awake to this moment? Or do you feel something else? Do you feel constricted, frustrated, angry?

It may seem strange to consciously focus on the negative. But it's worth remembering that at a subconscious level, favoring the negative is what the mind does all the time. As was discussed in the chapter titled "Understanding Our Set Point: The Biological Challenge of Being Human," our natural impulse is to dwell on potential threats to our social survival—on thoughts such as *I hate the way I look right now, I don't want to be doing this,* or *I need more money, time, love.*

Now let's explore the opposite of this set-point-driven biological tendency. Take a moment to write down three things in your life that you feel grateful for. These could be big things: your health, your romantic partner, or your children. Or they could be small: the delicious meal you just ate, the feeling of the wind in your hair, or the fact that you currently have a roof over your head.

1. _____

2. _____

3. _____

Now take fifteen to thirty seconds to appreciate and savor each of these gifts.

Check in with yourself again. Do you feel different than before? Do you feel more awake to this moment, more at peace, more joyful, happier?

If you felt a subtle change in your mind-set or even your physical awareness after this exercise, you are not alone. You are experiencing a shift that springs from the deepest levels of your neural anatomy. By consciously appreciating the good, we activate neural pathways that open the door to a deeper experience of wellbeing.

This isn't just speculation. Robert Emmons and Michael McCullough, two of the pioneers in the field of gratitude research, examined the effects of this very practice. They divided participants into several groups. One group spent ten weeks writing daily about hassles or irritants. Another wrote about events that affected them. The final group spent ten weeks writing down the things they were grateful for.

The results were astonishing. The consistent practice of gratitude had powerful effects on all aspects of wellbeing. Those in the gratitude group had a more positive attitude toward their life circumstances, exercised more, and reported fewer physical symptoms associated with headaches and other chronic health issues.[4]

This probably isn't the first time that you have heard about the beneficial effects of gratitude, and you have no doubt experienced them firsthand: while watching the sunset, tucking your child into bed, or sitting down to a meal with your family. The Gratitude practice will help you go beyond the occasional unexpected experience of feeling thankful for your life. Training this powerful skill turns gratitude into a gateway to a better life.

WHAT IT IS

We tend to talk about gratitude as a way of expressing our thankfulness—for a meal, an event, or an act of kindness. Following the lead of researchers in the field of positive psychology, we define gratitude more broadly: as the conscious appreciation of any aspect of our life experience. Sonja Lyubomirsky offers a poetic description:

> *It is wonder; it is appreciation; it is looking at the bright side of a setback; it is fathoming abundance; it is thanking someone in your life; it is thanking God; it is "counting blessings." It is savoring; it is not taking things for granted; it is coping; it is present-oriented.*[5]

Gratitude is the easiest and most efficient way to shift our set-point-driven state of mind. It's the ultimate shortcut to wellbeing. Fifteen seconds of savoring something you are grateful for can transform your perspective on life, turn problems into possibilities and irritation into curiosity. And like all three of the Be practices, gratitude is something you can do any time, anywhere. The challenge and real benefit comes from training the skill to become second nature so that you naturally savor gratitude throughout the day.

Jack, a former family business owner and a LIFE XT coach, describes a lifelong negative pattern that changed when he developed a daily habit of gratitude:

> *I used to focus on the "specks on the wall" of my life. Things that I didn't have (cooler job, bigger house) or wanted more of (money, power). I was keeping score in a game that didn't add up to what I really valued in life—my family, close connections with friends, and a job that was aligned with my purpose. I began to notice how often I focused on mostly the negative stuff. I developed a daily habit of gratitude and started keeping a gratitude journal. Now, when I begin to think about the specks, I shift to gratitude, and it completely changes my day. My best shift move, though, is to extend the feeling of gratitude and savor these moments by closing my eyes and taking a deep breath. It has transformed my life.*

We all have our own version of Jack's "specks on the wall." Without gratitude, we focus on these life imperfections; in fact they often become all that we can see. Gratitude gives us a bigger perspective. We may still see the imperfections—the specks in our lives—but we also recognize the blessings that surround them.

Ram Dass, a former Harvard psychologist and an acclaimed spiritual teacher, uses the analogy of a picture of the sky to illustrate this shift in perspective. If you have a photograph of the sky that is cropped in tight on a small gray cloud, that's all you can see. Everything looks dark and colorless. But if you zoom out and see the sky from a larger perspective, you begin to see that the cloud is surrounded by blue sky.[6] That's the shift in perspective you can access through gratitude.

To help you turn gratitude into a habit, you will use an everyday cue as your reminder: sitting down to eat a meal. Each time you eat with friends, family, or by yourself, you will use Notice-Shift-Rewire to shift your attention to gratitude. You will notice the things for which you are grateful and savor the felt experience of the gratitude shift. When you master this act of savoring—of staying with your experience of appreciation—you create new neural pathways and begin experiencing a positive shift in your outlook on life.

WHY IT WORKS

Like all the LIFE XT practices, gratitude is an age-old practice. The spiritual traditions of both East and West talk about gratitude as an essential act of appreciation for the divine. The Quran states, "Eat of the good things that We have provided for you, and be grateful to God, if it is Him that you worship."[7] The Christian tradition offers, in the Book of Timothy, "God created foods to be received with thanksgiving by those who believe and know the truth."[8] In Buddhist texts, gratitude is seen as cultivating kindness and virtue: "The worthy person is grateful and mindful of benefits done to him. This gratitude, this mindfulness, is congenial to the best people."[9]

For our purposes though, the most helpful historical discussion of gratitude arises from the writings of the ancient Greek Stoic philosopher Epictetus, a former slave. His philosophy is complex and covers a wide span of intellectual terrain. Yet you can boil down much of his thinking on how to live a better life to a simple contemporary slogan: Happiness is an inside job.

It sounds simple enough. But Epictetus noticed that most of us follow the opposite strategy. We go through our days desperately trying to control our external circumstances. We want more love from our partner, more money from our job, more time in our schedule, more respect from our colleagues, and on and on. Simply put—we try to find happiness outside of ourselves. And rarely, if ever, does the world fully cooperate with our wishes.

So Epictetus offered a different strategy, what Dartmouth University classics professor Margaret Graver calls a strategy of "emotional adjustment."[10] The basic idea is this: It's far easier to reshape and adjust our inner world than the outer world. It's more effective to adjust our beliefs about money than to instantly make huge sums of money. It's more practical to adjust our beliefs about relationships than to find a perfect partner without a single flaw. So when it comes to gratitude, Epictetus declares, "He is a wise man who does not grieve for the things which he has not, but rejoices for those which he has."[11]

This is the core insight behind the Gratitude practice. When we grieve for the things we don't have, we suffer. When we rejoice for the things we do have, we experience contentment. This might sound like the path to complacency—to giving up our aspirations for a better, healthier, more prosperous life. But it's often the opposite. Our grief for the things we wish we had can leave us wallowing in envy, bitterness, and self-pity. When we make this gratitude adjustment and no longer resist what is, we unleash great stores of energy that we can use to engage more effectively in the world around us.

Fast-forward a couple of thousand years from Epictetus and company, and we now have the scientific evidence to show that this ancient wisdom holds a whole host of benefits for emotional and physical wellbeing. Gratitude diminishes anxiety, depression, and other signs of psychological unease while simultaneously cultivating appreciation and contentment.

How does gratitude work? As we learned in the chapter on set points, our brain sorts all our memories and experiences into two piles of judgments: memories that incite approach (attachment) and those that incite aversion (resistance). The problem is that not all memories and experiences are stored with the same level of priority. The brain tends to prioritize the negative. As we learned in the set point chapter, the brain is "like Velcro for negative experiences and Teflon for positive ones."[12] Traumatic experiences—car accidents, heartbreak, or intense fear—carve deep grooves in the neural structures of the brain. This is why walking by the park bench where your last breakup occurred can leave you in tears or why the anniversary of an accident brings up painful memories. Meanwhile, positive experiences—getting married, the birth of a child, and other major accomplishments—tend to have only fleeting effects on our happiness. If we don't consciously savor these experiences, they quickly fade away.

The brain's Velcro-like attachment to bad experiences reinforces the negativity bias of the set point mind. It ensures that we spend the bulk of our mental energy ruminating on regrets, resentments, and fears, rather than contemplating moments of bliss and elation. Recent research, however, has also found there is an easy antidote to this negative spiral: gratitude. Even though our brains are naturally attracted to negative memories, *gratitude* allows us to amplify the positive—to create more powerful and vivid positive memories and, in turn, lasting changes to the brain.

In fact, the research of Barbara Fredrickson, a psychologist at the University of North Carolina, has shown that gratitude "broadens and builds" the brain's capacity to overcome negative states.[13] In the absence of gratitude, the mind closes in on a small handful of possibilities. Gratitude expands the field by "widening the array of thoughts and actions that come to mind."[14] If you feel frustration while sitting in traffic, for example, gratitude helps broaden your experience. You can begin to notice the changing leaves on the trees, relax into your breath, or use the delay as an opportunity to really listen to your favorite album.

This shift isn't merely psychological. Evidence from neuroscience suggests that this practice extends deep into the neural pathways of the brain. Richard Davidson notes, "From everything we know about the brain circuitry underlying these components it's a good bet that wellbeing therapy [the expression of gratitude for self and others] strengthens the prefrontal cortex."[15]

As psychologists continue to explore the causal mechanisms behind gratitude, one thing is clear. Gratitude offers extensive benefits of wellbeing, including:

- *Increased optimism.* Research demonstrates that the practice correlates to an increase in the experience of positive emotions and reduction of negative ones.[16]
- *Reduced stress and anxiety in times of crisis.* In studies following the September 11 attacks on the World Trade Center and elsewhere, Fredrickson found that the practice of gratitude diminished the intensity and frequency of traumatic memories.[17]

- *Enhanced physical health.* Gratitude improves both cardio-vascular health and also the quality of our sleep. Researchers have found that by practicing gratitude, we get more sleep, fall asleep more easily, and feel better when we wake up.[18]
- *Improved relationships.* Emmons and McCullough theorize that gratitude within relationships can create a kind of "upward spiral." As we become more grateful for our friends and family, we treat them with more kindness and respect.

The evidence that practicing gratitude enhances wellbeing is overwhelming. But remember, the ultimate proof isn't what the ancients said or what the latest study concluded. It's how you feel when you integrate the regular practice of gratitude into your daily life.

HOW TO DEVELOP THIS SKILL

Habit 5: Gratitude

How to do it: To build this daily habit, we recommend that you use meals as your cue to Notice-Shift-Rewire to gratitude. Notice each time you sit down to eat. Shift by redirecting your attention to gratitude. If you are alone, take a moment to think about a few things that you are grateful for in that moment. If you are with friends, family, or coworkers, you might tell them about your LIFE XT Gratitude practice and see if they are open to sharing what they are grateful for. Then give each person the opportunity to express one thing that

(continued on next page)

they are grateful for in that moment. Rewire by taking a few seconds to savor your feelings of gratitude.

Of course, LIFE XT isn't unique in using meals as a cue for experiencing gratitude. This practice runs throughout many religious traditions and even shows up during national holidays like Thanksgiving. It's a way of honoring our good fortune. By expressing our appreciation for these basic necessities of life, we shift the mind from stories about what we wish we had to the present reality of what we already do have. For more practical tips and strategies for building the habit of gratitude, see the chapter "How to Practice Life Cross Training" at the end of the book.

Beyond Dining: Gratitude in the Rest of Life

We recommend you start by using meals as your cue to experience gratitude. As this practice becomes a habit, you can incorporate gratitude in other areas of your life. Like Presence, this is a practice that you can do anytime, anywhere: watching a summer storm, walking with a friend, or even waiting at the dentist's office to get your teeth cleaned.

Gratitude is also particularly powerful in the workplace. This one practice can transform the culture of an office. A statement of appreciation—"I loved your talk yesterday" or "I appreciate your passion for your work"—can transform workplace relationships into moments of genuine connection.

To experience this shift in almost any situation, use the inner technology of Notice-Shift-Rewire.

Step 1: Notice

When it comes to gratitude, you can notice in two ways. The first is noticing the negative. You probably go through much of the day cycling through one negative thought after another, usually without even knowing it. It's easy to get caught in stories about what is wrong with your job, your marriage, or your health—to get lost in a sea of *in*gratitude. However, when you notice your negative thoughts, you can use them as a trigger to make the shift to gratitude.

Chad, a successful screenwriter for a popular television series, describes his experience of noticing the negative:

> *After spending ten hours at work, I walk in the door and see every-*
> *thing that's wrong. The dogs haven't been taken out, the sink is full*
> *of dirty dishes, and we're out of my favorite soda. I can't help but*
> *feel irritated and angry. But I am learning that if I can just catch*
> *myself, if I can see that I'm lost in negative thoughts, everything*
> *changes. I take a deep breath, think about one thing that I'm grate-*
> *ful for in that moment, and I become a much better person to be*
> *around.*

The second technique is noticing the positive. Why draw our attention to the good thoughts and emotions that arise organically? By noticing the positive, you can amplify your experience of these positive thoughts and emotions, and in so doing, balance the negative bias of the set point mind. Our day-to-day lives are filled with positive noticing cues, large and small: a big win at work, the feeling of being at peace on a long walk, your dog greeting you at the door at the end of a long day, or finding that your partner has done your laundry for you.

Step 2: Shift

Shifting to gratitude is straightforward. It's the practice of redirecting your attention toward gratitude. If you find yourself dwelling on the negative, think of something you are grateful for in this moment. It might be the warmth of the sun coming through your window. It might be the fact that you have food in your fridge or that you have so many amazing friends and family members.

Step 3: Rewire

With the Gratitude practice, we place a special emphasis on Rewire. Many Gratitude practices fall short of this essential step. And yet savoring—taking a moment to enjoy the experience of gratitude—plays a key role in placing these positive experiences into long-term memory and turning gratitude into a daily habit.

When noticing the negative, shift to gratitude, and then take as little as fifteen to thirty seconds to feel this new habit seeping into your body and mind. Feel the sensations that arise when you experience appreciation. Stay with it and feel it so deeply that you create a strong imprint in your brain.

Try it now. Think of one thing that you are grateful for. Once you experience the gratitude shift, take fifteen seconds to savor the feeling. Stay with the experience and notice the physiological changes in your body.

Sharon, a successful entrepreneur, explains how shifting to gratitude helped her during a moment of crisis in her life:

> *After my mother's death and the illness of my son, I sought a therapist's help to deal with the ensuing depression and anxiety. Seeking to interrupt my pattern of negative thought and worry, this time about my son's illness, she asked me to write down as many positive*

things about him as I could think up. As I warmed to the exercise, the list became lengthy and more important, as I began to let these positive attributes sink in deeply, my anxiety about his health virtually disappeared, replaced by overwhelming love and enjoyment of him as an individual.

For Sharon, shifting her attention to gratitude and savoring the good transformed anxiety into love and appreciation.

Joyfully Share

One of the most effective ways to share your experience of gratitude is by expressing your appreciation to others.[19] Most of us go through life only occasionally telling the people we love most just how much we care about them. The shift here is exchanging some of that energy—tell others what it is you appreciate about them. Tell someone you love why they are amazing. Tell your friends why you love having them in your life. Tell the clerk who carries your purchases to the car how grateful you are for his help. After each appreciation, check in and notice how you feel. Savor this feeling. Rejoice in the smiles that are returned to you. Tune in to how your own smile feels.

The more you Notice-Shift-Rewire to gratitude, the more you will experience a sense of inner richness.

WHAT TO EXPECT

You can expect to feel some benefit from your Gratitude practice almost instantly. The powerful effects of gratitude arise the moment you begin taking in the good.

While its benefits are instant, you can also expect to experience a few changes in your Gratitude practice as you first develop and then refine the habit. As with presence, the first stage in developing gratitude is to develop the habit. During this period, you will need to exert conscious effort to remember to Notice-Shift-Rewire to gratitude each day. For example, as you practice gratitude at meals, you must overcome a lifetime of habits that direct the unconscious flow of your actions. The momentum of habit will lead you to dive into your meal without considering all that you are grateful for.

So during this stage, the key is to remember. We offer a number of tips and strategies for remembering in the chapter "How to Practice Life Cross Training" at the end of the book, but we have found that two strategies work best. First, get your friends and family members involved. Then when you sit down to a meal with them, you can help each other remember. Second, if all else fails, put a small sticker with the word *NSR* or *Gratitude* on the upper corner of your place mat. This will give you a visual reminder each time you eat at home. Within a month, practicing gratitude over meals will become a habit.

As you develop the habits of noticing and shifting, remember that the key to the LIFE XT practice of Gratitude is to focus on rewiring the felt experience. This act of savoring is another counter-habitual move. Left unchecked, our tendency is to treat gratitude like another item on our daily to-do list. We do it and then move on to the next thing as quickly as possible. Try to interrupt this impulse. Instead of diving into your salad the moment you finish expressing gratitude, give yourself a little space—just a moment—to savor the experience.

After about a month of consistent practice, you will have made it through the period of habit formation. You should now notice that it takes almost no mental energy to notice each time you sit down to a meal.

As the habit deepens, you will also start to notice the experience of gratitude popping up at random moments throughout the day. You may find yourself extending your practice of Notice-Shift-Rewire beyond meals: as you open your email inbox, at the end of meetings, or before you fall asleep each night. You may also notice unconscious expressions of gratitude pouring out of you during the course of ordinary conversation. You might find yourself talking more about your gratitude for the weather, for your family, for your work, and for your health, often without even knowing it.

Above all, you will find your mind shifting in the ways Epictetus described thousands of years ago: You will think less about what you wish you had and more about all that you do have. Nate's ninety-five-year old grandma Hilda arrived at this rich insight after a lifetime of her own gratitude practice. As she explained to Nate one sunny August afternoon, "Gratitude—that's something I try to keep in my mind all the time. Be grateful for what I already have, not what I think I would like to have, just what I already have right here, right now."

Hilda's wise words point to the deep connection between the Gratitude and Presence practices. Gratitude for what we "already have right here, right now" also takes us out of mind wandering and brings us back to this moment.

PRACTICE 6: COMPASSION

Getting strangled rarely brings out the best in people.

But that's exactly what happened one day when Mahatma Gandhi visited a small village in India. It was an ordinary town on an ordinary day. Gandhi stood peacefully in the center of a busy town square filled with the shouts of shopkeepers and the bustle of a crowded marketplace.

Then something unexpected happened. Eknath Easwaran, Gandhi's biographer, captured the moment: "a notoriously fierce communal agitator came up to Gandhi in front of a crowd of paralyzed onlookers, put his hands around Gandhi's slender throat, and began choking the life out of him."[1]

We all know that Gandhi led an Indian independence movement based on the idea of *ahimsa*, the Sanskrit word for nonviolence. But this act of aggression presented the ultimate challenge to his core principle of compassion. How would he react in the face of violence?

With the hands of a fanatic wrapped around his neck, what did Gandhi do? He shifted to compassion. He didn't fight back, nor did he resist, nor did he become paralyzed by fear. In the words of Easwaran, "there was not even a flicker of hostility in his eyes, not a word of protest. He yielded himself completely to the flood of love within him."[2]

This counter-instinctual move shocked everyone, including the crazed man clutching Gandhi's neck. In fact, he was so shocked that his violent rage melted like ice in the hot Indian sun. As the story goes, "the man broke down like a little child," writes Easwaran, "and fell sobbing at his feet."[3]

This story illustrates what it looks like to master the skill of compassion. Like an Olympian who spends years training for a single jump, swim, or sprint, Gandhi spent a lifetime training for such a moment. "I hold myself incapable of hating any being on earth," Gandhi explained. "By a long course of prayerful discipline, I have ceased for over forty years to hate anyone."[4]

Gandhi's words point to an essential truth: We all have the capacity to employ more compassion in our lives. And when we turn this virtue into a practice, we live differently. Without compassion, our days can leave us feeling reactive, irritated, and angry. The world becomes our enemy and stress our constant companion. With compassion, we feel more empathy, ease, and understanding. The world becomes friendlier and everyday stressors begin to lose their grip over us.

WHAT IT IS

We think of compassion as arising from a simple formula:

EMPATHY + LOVE = COMPASSION

Empathy gives us the ability to understand the viewpoints and feelings of others. While empathy is important, it falls short of compassion. You can *understand* the feelings of a friend, a relative, or an acquaintance while still feeling bitterness or resentment toward them. Compassion adds love to the equation. It arises when we combine our ability to empathize with others with a heartfelt sense of love.[5]

In its ideal form, compassion has no boundaries. It goes beyond extending loving-kindness to our inner circle of friends, family members, and other loved ones. Compassion is the art of loving all beings—even those who would seek to do us harm. It's also about opening to love ourselves, even those dark and hard to reach corners of our being.

Like gratitude, the practice of compassion is something all of us have encountered. You have no doubt experienced it from others directed toward you: in a moment of crisis or following the death of a loved one. You have also likely experienced this state of empathetic love toward others and at times toward yourself.

We all understand the importance and benefits of compassion. Yet in the midst of everyday life, compassion is one of the most difficult states to access. Not that presence and gratitude are easy, but while you are standing in an hour-long line at the Department of Motor Vehicles, it's easier to follow your breath or think about gratitude than it is to feel deep love for the people ahead of you in line or for those working the counter.

While we are juggling the many demands of modern life, it's also easy to simply forget to access this powerful state. We often overlook the needs of others, not out of any feeling of ill will but because we are just too busy or distracted to make a connection. This is the challenge that we all face in building the habit of compassion. While we may want to feel more compassion for others, the busyness of our schedules—and our own minds—distracts us. The fast pace of life often leaves us with a gap between our desire to live with compassion and our actions toward others.

The Compassion practice gives you a way to rewire the impulse for caring into an everyday habit—to become more aware of opportunities to extend compassion to others. When you make this shift, your daily life opens to moments of grace and profound joy.

Try it right now. As a thought experiment, think of a public figure—a celebrity, pro athlete, or political figure—who angers you or whom you deeply disagree with. If you are having trouble, just think of the most radical person you can identify on the opposite end of the political spectrum. Close your eyes and bring this person's image to mind. What are the sensations arising in your body? What are the thoughts looping through your mind? Use this feeling of irritation as a cue to Notice-Shift-Rewire. Now shift—spend fifteen to thirty seconds feeling deep compassion for this person. If it helps, repeat the phrase "May you be well and happy" while picturing them in your mind.

Now check in again. Do you feel any different? If you do, you just experienced firsthand the shift of compassion. With a little practice, your ability to Notice-Shift-Rewire to compassion will become second nature, and the actual compassion shift will become richer and longer lasting. You will notice less tension, anger, frustration, and irritation. As you become more open, kindhearted, and generous, your friends and family may also notice a difference in you. Chances are, you will even see this shift reflected back, as your friends, family, and coworkers become less reactive, defensive, and irritated in your presence.

To turn compassion into a daily habit, you will use an everyday cue to help you notice: leaving your home (house, apartment, dorm room, etc.). Each time you walk out your door, your practice will be to develop the habit of experiencing deep compassion for the people you will encounter as you head out to work, to school, to the store, or to your child's baseball game. The ultimate goal is to train the skill of noticing—of becoming aware of the limitless opportunities for living with compassion.

WHY IT WORKS

Gandhi's idea of compassion arose from the powerful texts of the Hindu tradition, but compassion isn't unique to any single philosophical or spiritual tradition. Almost every religion advocates a similar practice of shifting from hatred to love.

In most traditions, this shift toward compassion is said to work by dissolving fear and hatred. The Buddha states in the Dhammapada, "Hatreds never cease through hatred in this world; through love alone they cease. This is an eternal law."[6]

This shift toward compassion is also described as radical—as an extreme act of love. It's not simply about loving your family, your friends, or your fellow citizens. It's about extending love to all beings—even those who do not mean you well.

We see this idea emerge in the *Tao Te Ching*. In Lao-tzu's words (as translated by Stephen Mitchell):

The Master . . . is good to people who are good.
She is also good to people who aren't good.
This is true goodness.[7]

For many of us, the idea of being good to those who aren't good sounds unfair. We tend to love conditionally. We love those who are good to us. We love those who share our beliefs, our political party, or our nationality. But when it comes to those who don't—to those who "aren't good"—we tend to retreat into resentment and hatred, creating distance rather than making a connection.

Compassion, however, is the act of shifting beyond this learned human impulse. Jesus declares in the Book of Matthew, "You have heard that it was said, 'You shall love your neighbor and hate your enemy.' But I say to you, Love your enemies and pray for those who persecute you, so that you may be sons of your Father who is in heaven" (5:43–45).

All of the traditions converge on the idea that to be compassionate is to offer our greatest love to *all* beings. In the midst of everyday life, this idea has remarkable implications. Consider that ex-spouse, boyfriend, or girlfriend who stirs strong negative emotions within you. Consider the driver who waits for what seems like an hour to take a left turn in front of you. Consider the people in your life who have caused you the most harm. Each of these situations evokes an emotional response that serves as an opportunity to Notice-Shift-Rewire to compassion.

Compassion is the act of forgiving and loving through all the layers of judgment, attachment, and resistance that arise in the presence of those who cause you difficulty. You can go through an entire lifetime judging the behavior of these people, attaching to your feelings of resentment, and resisting the idea that you can love what seems unlovable. Compassion opens the door to living with a more loving, less stressful life experience.

Of course, living in the moment-to-moment state of this kind of radical compassion isn't easy. It doesn't happen overnight. Gandhi understood the great difficulty of living in this state. So he advised his followers to "start where you are . . . If you can't love the Viceroy, or Sir Winston Churchill," he would say, "start with your wife, or your husband, or your children. Try to put their welfare first and your own last every minute of the day, and let the circle of your love expand from there."[8]

Recent discoveries in neuroscience reveal that the power of compassion goes beyond the spiritual realm. As with the Presence and Gratitude practices, the Compassion practice also changes the brain in ways that expand our overall experience of wellbeing.

Forgiveness

Forgiveness is a central aspect of compassion. Think of it as compassion extended toward past harms. The twentieth-century German political theorist Hannah Arendt describes the act of forgiveness as the primary gateway to finding freedom from past suffering. Forgiveness, she says, "frees from its consequences both the one who forgives and the one who is forgiven."

The first step in forgiveness is to say that, while the actions of the other person may not be okay, you will not let these actions destroy you. The second, more challenging step is to find compassion for the other person. When you succeed in making this shift, you will have created a radical change in your inner world that may also change the events and circumstances of your outer world.

Richard Davidson has led the way in documenting the powerful effects of compassion on the brain. He examined what happens when experienced meditators like Matthieu Ricard shifted from an ordinary state to compassion meditation.

Davidson asked these meditators to start by envisioning those they cared most about—their partners, friends, or family. The goal was to feel the deep sense of altruistic love for these people and then extend the circle. By the end of the practice, subjects ended up extending compassion beyond their inner circles to all beings (the very same practice you will learn at the end of the chapter).[9]

When Davidson's team examined the brain activation patterns of this group, they noticed huge increases in gamma activity and neural synchronicity. As Davidson remarked, "During [compassion] meditation gamma activity was greater than had ever been reported in the scientific literature."[10] This is important because gamma waves are associated with the feeling of blessings, contentment, and extremely high levels of cognitive functioning.

While the results were impressive, Davidson's team also wanted to know whether these findings translated to those with no formal compassion meditation practice. Led by Helen Weng, a graduate student at the Davidson lab, researchers used fMRI to measure the brain activity of participants viewing images of human suffering. Participants were given thirty minutes per day of training in compassion meditation, and the researchers took measurements at the beginning of the study and two weeks later. They found that the brain activity of the subject group had shifted radically. As Davidson observed, "Those who had undergone training in compassion meditation showed striking changes in brain function, particularly in the amygdala."[11] The amygdala is the section of the brain that controls our fight-or-flight response. Reduced activation in this region indicated that compassion meditation had enabled participants to feel less distress. The subjects also displayed increased altruistic behavior and increased activation in the regions of the brain involved in social cognition and emotional regulation.[12]

It's easy to get lost in the details of these scientific studies. But the big insight here is that by practicing compassion meditation for a short time, you positively change your brain. With continued practice, this leads to experiencing an ongoing state of compassion in your life and creates a powerful virtuous cycle. Compassion helps you live with a more positive outlook, which in turn helps you become more loving and empathetic toward others.

HOW TO DEVELOP THIS SKILL

To train this skill, the Compassion practice gives you two robust tools. The first practice uses Notice-Shift-Rewire to build a daily habit of compassion. The second practice is a form of meditation designed to cultivate the skill of compassion, a technique called loving-kindness, or *metta*.

Beyond the Front Door: Compassion in the Rest of Life

Habit 6: Compassion

How to do it: To build this daily habit, use leaving your home each day as your cue to Notice-Shift-Rewire to compassion. Notice each time you leave, whether you are headed to work or just headed to the store to pick up groceries. Shift by redirecting your attention to compassion. As you walk out the door, think of all the people you will come in contact with that day, and take a moment to feel compassion toward them. You can do this by flooding your body with a feeling of love for these people or by thinking to yourself, "May everyone I come in contact with today be happy." Rewire by taking a few seconds to savor this flood of loving-kindness.

Why practice compassion as you leave the home each day? Leaving the house is a key moment of transition. It represents a shift from a space that you control (your home) to a space that you have almost no control over (the office, the highway, the subway car, and so on). By experiencing compassion at this threshold to the outer world, you will improve your ability to handle the challenging situations that may arise along the way: parking tickets, reckless drivers, irritating coworkers, and on and on. For more practical tips and strategies for building the habit of compassion, see the chapter "How to Practice Life Cross Training" at the end of the book.

The primary Compassion practice is to Notice-Shift-Rewire to compassion as you leave the house each day. As you walk out your door, you will begin to prioritize the experience of compassion at the start of each day. You will be more likely to feel love and kindness, rather than irritation and anxiety, toward those whom you encounter.

In the midst of your everyday life, you can also use the felt sense of negative emotions as a powerful trigger for shifting to compassion. When you feel a difficult emotion, use it as a signal to shift. Potent emotional triggers include irritation, anger, frustration, sadness, and fear. If these triggers involve internal insecurities, they can provide a powerful opportunity for shifting toward compassion for yourself. In these moments and throughout your day, here's how you can begin to experience more compassion.

Step 1: Notice

The first step is to notice the absence of compassion toward yourself. When it comes to compassion toward ourselves, most of us have an internal critic whose presence signals the need to shift. This inner critic takes on infinite forms. It might tell you, *You should be better, You're lazy,* or *You're going to fail.* Notice these messages.

When it comes to noticing a lack of compassion for others, look for the same messages, projected onto other people. Your inner judge is likely to think things like *That guy is messy, She's full of herself,* or *He's too needy.* Notice these judgments. Notice the natural tendency of the set point mind to view others with a negative bias. Notice how your thoughts distance you from the other person.

Step 2: Shift

When you notice this absence of compassion, shift. Shifting doesn't require that you meditate for thirty minutes. It doesn't require that you hang up the phone or leave the meeting you are in. You can make this shift instantly in the midst of your daily life.

The shift is to simply acknowledge the thought. See it for what it is: a thought. Take a second to feel the physical reaction in your body associated with this thought. Take a breath and release it. Now redirect your attention and thoughts to a compassionate or positive feeling toward the person(s) or situation. It can also be helpful to repeat in your mind a phrase like *May you be at ease and happy* or one of the other phrases in the compassion meditation later in the chapter.

Shifting to compassion when you think about your "annoying neighbor," "nitpicky spouse," or "arrogant coworker" can be counter-habitual and will likely feel strange at first. But as you develop this skill, it gets easier and more instinctual. Take a moment to try it right now.

Step 3: Rewire

The final step is to take a brief moment—just fifteen to thirty seconds—to savor the feeling of compassion. Let this felt experience that compassion evokes in your mind and body sink in. Notice the difference between this experience of compassion and the experience of anger, irritation, or contempt. Encode this experience deep in the neural connections of the brain; allow the neurons of compassion that fire together to begin to wire together. Live in a state of kindness and compassion.

Kaley, an executive coach, tells us about the challenge of incorporating this practice into her life while traveling for work:

> *Because I travel multiple times per week for work, airports are like the double-black diamonds of compassion. I notice my judgment*

everywhere. People should know how to navigate TSA, the agents should be doing their jobs more efficiently, the others on my plane shouldn't talk so loudly or so much. Now I try to use travel as a time to practice compassion. By starting with kindness, I have a lot more patience, can use my experience to be helpful instead of harsh, and it usually makes the experience much more enjoyable.

Kaley's story shows that you can practice compassion anytime, anywhere. A regular traveler like Kaley uses airports as her cue. You already know many of your own triggers for impatience and aggravation. By recognizing these and creating your own cues for compassion, you can build space around your practice and put yourself in a state where you are available to Notice-Shift-Rewire.

We have found that the checkout line is another powerful place for compassion. Instead of feeling impatient with the person in front of you who can't quite figure out how to scan his credit card, notice your irritation and make the shift to compassion. Instead of feeling rushed when it's your turn to pay, take a moment to put yourself in the shoes of the store clerk. Direct loving-kindness toward her as you pay. It will change your day—and possibly hers as well.

Compassion Through Meditation

The second Compassion practice is a new way of meditating. By now you have started developing a focused-attention practice of meditation, in which you direct your awareness to the sensations of breath. Compassion meditation can change the very structure of the brain in just two weeks.[13]

This meditation consists of reciting a short repeated phrase while cycling our focus toward the following people and groups:

- A loved one
- Yourself
- A difficult person
- All beings

To begin, it might be useful to review tips on meditation in the chapters "Practice 1: Meditation" and "How to Practice Life Cross Training." We also recommend downloading the guided compassion meditation from the LIFE XT website or any other site or app that offers guided practices.

Start by sitting with a straight spine, and take a few minutes to observe your breathing.

A Loved One

Begin by picturing a loved one. It might be a parent, a child, or your spouse. As you focus on this image, recite the following words:

May you be filled with loving-kindness.
May you be safe from inner and outer dangers.
May you be well in body and mind.
May you be at ease and happy.[14]

Feel the waves of love and kindness pulsating through your body as you imagine your loved one. Feel the depth of your wish for them to experience love and to be free from suffering.

After several minutes, take another brief meditative rest by returning your attention to your breathing.

Self

The next step is to turn inward, to yourself. As you continue to breathe smoothly, recite the following phrases inwardly:

May I be filled with loving-kindness.
May I be safe from inner and outer dangers.
May I be well in body and mind.
May I be at ease and happy.[15]

As you recite these words you might picture yourself either as you are today or as a child. Allow loving-kindness to flood every part of you, even those dark corners of your being that are difficult to accept.

After a few minutes, take a brief meditative rest by returning to the observation of your breathing.

Difficult People

The next step is to expand loving-kindness beyond those who are easy to love. It is to practice the art of loving the people in your life who have cheated you, betrayed you, or caused you pain. Picture one such person and then repeat the same mantra as before:

May you be filled with loving-kindness.
May you be safe from inner and outer dangers.
May you be well in body and mind.
May you be at ease and happy.[16]

In this stage of the meditation, you may encounter some difficult emotions. You may feel waves of resentment, anger, or fear arise. Let that be okay. See if you can experience deep love while simultaneously allowing these waves of emotion to move through. Remember that this person has also suffered. You might picture him or her as a child.

After several minutes, take another brief meditative rest by returning your attention to your breathing.

Love All Beings

The final stage is to extend loving-kindness to all beings. Picture the earth from space. As you visualize this image, recite the very same mantra:

> *May all beings be filled with loving-kindness.*
> *May all beings be safe from inner and outer dangers.*
> *May all beings be well in body and mind.*
> *May all beings be at ease and happy.*[17]

Try to feel the suffering of all of humanity and sentient beings, while simultaneously experiencing the waves of love and compassion that flow out of your mind and body. Direct every ounce of your attention toward the experience of love. Imagine that you alone have the power to eradicate hunger, violence, and suffering through the intensity of your focus on loving-kindness.

After several minutes, return your attention to your breath. When you are ready, open your eyes and return to your day.

Grant, a participant in the LIFE XT program at a digital media agency, shares his early observations of compassion meditation:

> *I started meditating two years ago, and as I scrolled through all of the guided meditations on my app, I intentionally avoided com-*

passion meditations. At the time I thought they were cheesy. The idea of having compassion toward those that were hurtful was too New Age for me. Then one day I decided to just try a compassion meditation. About halfway through, I began sobbing right there in my living room. The idea of feeling true compassion for myself, my children, my coworkers, even my ex-wife, opened up a whole new area of my heart in such a profound way. I am still growing in this area, and it is not always easy, but this practice has forever changed me. I have noticed that the level of anger I feel toward others in stressful situations has decreased dramatically, and I have become more relaxed with myself when conflict arises in my life.

Many people share Grant's experience. They underestimate the power of this practice. But experiencing love and empathy for the people in your life has the power to radically change your relationship to yourself and others.

A Quick Tip: Start Slow

As with any kind of training, we encourage you to start slowly and work your way up to the later steps. Mingyur Rinpoche says of compassion meditation, "Training in loving-kindness and compassion has to be undertaken gradually."[18] As you begin exploring compassion meditation, remember this advice: You are your own best guide. Pay close attention to how you feel, as you should with all the practices in LIFE XT. Let your experience be your ultimate guide.

WHAT TO EXPECT

The Compassion practice gives you the tools to rewire your brain and change your life. Like the other Being and Doing practices, this change happens both rapidly and gradually. After just one sitting of compassion meditation, you will notice a change in the way you feel. You will feel more love for yourself and others; you will feel greater ease and more at peace.

For many people, however, the Compassion practice is less intuitive than one like Gratitude. During the initial stage of habit formation, you may encounter one or more of the following challenges:

- *Thinking this seems too "soft."* Let's face it, it's hard to talk about sending waves of love toward yourself and others without sounding "out there." For many people, this stigma keeps them from experiencing the powerful benefits of compassion. If you run into this challenge, see if you can simply notice the judgments that arise in your mind: *This is weird*, *It's too 1960s Haight-Ashbury*, or *I'm not one of those people*. See them as thoughts (you could even do inquiry on them) and then return to the practice. Don't let the softness of words like *love* and *empathy* keep you from experiencing wellbeing.

- *Feeling pity.* When you first start practicing compassion, it can be easy to fall into the trap of feeling sorry for other people. There's a subtle distinction between compassion and pity, and feeling sorry for others creates an unhelpful dynamic. If you walk by a homeless person, compassion isn't saying to yourself, *I feel sorry for that guy. I'm glad I'm not him*. Compassion works without judgment. It's the realization that, had it not been for your more fortunate circumstances, you could be him. To feel compassion is to love others simply because they are fellow beings.

- *Fearing of becoming too passive.* Some people worry that the practice of compassion could lead them to become passive and lose their drive to accomplish things and address problems. *If I'm all compassion, all the time,* they think, *then I'll lose motivation and people will walk all over me.* We have found that the opposite is true. When you live in a state of compassion, you free up energy that would otherwise go toward anger, irritation, and resentment. You can now direct this energy in far more productive ways. Compassion also doesn't preclude you from setting clear boundaries. You can Notice-Shift-Rewire and feel compassion toward a colleague who has been behaving badly while also expressing your disapproval or taking action to remedy the situation. Compassion allows you to do this from a place of love.

- *Having difficulty letting go.* The final challenge you may encounter is letting go of anger, irritation, and resentment. As you begin extending compassion to the difficult people in your life, you will almost inevitably encounter this challenge. In a strange way, resentment often feels safe. It's a form of self-protection. But it actually causes incredible suffering. If you can't let go, let that be okay. But if you can take this leap, you will notice a freeing shift in your life.

Once you move through these initial challenges and establish the habit of compassion through Notice-Shift-Rewire and compassion meditation, you will begin to enter a stage where compassion feels increasingly familiar and comforting. Don't expect to feel compassion all the time. But you will likely notice unexpected bursts of compassion arising more frequently as you go through your day. You might also notice that when you feel irritation or resentment, your mind feels less stuck. You are more likely to create the space to think, *How would this situation change if I felt compassion?*

If you are successful in extending compassion to yourself and to those who are causing you pain, you are likely to begin experiencing a profound transformation during this stage. This practice has the potential to heal lifelong patterns of anger and resentment. Eric reveals how compassion helped him radically shift his relationship with his father and stepmother

I spent much of my early life feeling anger toward my father and my stepmother. My father remarried when I was fourteen, shortly after my mother, whom I loved dearly, passed away. My relationship with my recently divorced stepmother, who was twenty years younger than my father and who came into a household that included three lost teenage boys, was strained from the start. She was possessive of my father's love and attention, and my brothers and I responded with feelings of sadness, resentment, helplessness, and anger.

After years of unhappiness, I slowly came to realize that holding on to my anger was not serving me in any way. Complaining about the situation offered little more than temporary relief from pain and usually left me feeling emptier and somewhat depressed. Over time (and without the benefit of LIFE XT), I cobbled together a rudimentary Compassion practice. To my own amazement, I learned to feel genuine empathy for my stepmother. I began to see that she had been doing the very best she could while faced with three resentful and sometimes wild teenage boys. This understanding set me free.

Today, after many years of practicing compassion for them, my relationship with both my father and stepmother is strong and full of affection, free from the drain of anger and resentment.

Eric's story is a reminder of the powerful impact of compassion. These feelings of anger, resentment, and bitterness diminish our sense of wellbeing. They can cause us to close down, put up internal barriers, and go numb. When you use these negative emotions as a trigger to experience compassion, however, you begin to feel a sense of aliveness and vibrancy.

The real power of this practice is that it extends far beyond each of us as individuals. As we become more loving and empathetic toward others, we create profound change in the world around us. When we move through the day with compassion, we enhance the lives of our friends, family members, coworkers, and the people we meet randomly throughout the day.

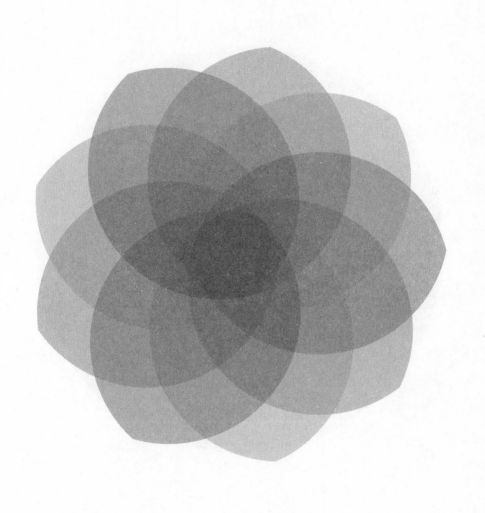

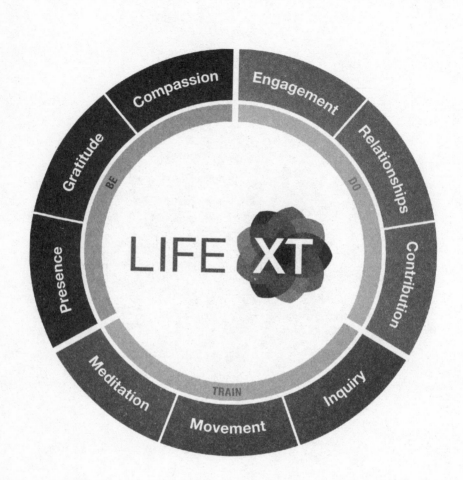

Give Your Gift to the World

You have now tasted the experience of being fully in the moment. The three habits of Presence, Gratitude, and Compassion have begun to shift your inner experience of life—helping you become more awake, aware, and present to each moment.

The final stage of LIFE XT shifts from the inner to the outer world, from being to doing. The aim of the LIFE XT program isn't to achieve one or the other. Rather, it's to find the balance between these two essential life virtues—to learn the art of *being* while *doing*. In everyday life, this balance occurs when we experience the richness of the three inner states of being while simultaneously staying engaged in our work, our relationships, and our community.

The Delight of Doing

Like being, doing can be seen as a spectrum running from actions that diminish wellbeing to those that enhance it—from surviving to thriving.

When we work so hard that we struggle to make it through each day, we live in the state of *survival*. It's not that we lack food, shelter, and other basic resources (though that could be the case).

It's that all of our effort is directed toward satisfying our own ever-expanding needs. Our experience becomes one of scarcity, relentless competition, and constantly satisfying our own needs.

SURVIVING	THRIVING	DOING
Scarcity	Abundance	
Self-interest	Contribution	
Workaholism	Balance	
Competition	Collaboration	
Stress	Flow	
Anxiety	Challenge	
Unease	Contentment	

The key shift of doing is from *surviving* to *thriving*. When we thrive, our workdays no longer feel like marathons. Rather than straining and struggling, we act with a sense of purpose and are fully engaged in our efforts. Most important, the goal of our work expands beyond mere survival. We're not solely concerned with our own needs. Instead, we work to give our maximum contribution to the world. The experience of thriving is the experience of abundance, collaboration, and making a positive impact on the world. *Thriving* is what happens when you give your fully actualized gift to the world.

Our contributions don't need to be grand or publicly celebrated. Few of us will come up with a cure for cancer or AIDS. Thriving can take many forms. Your gift to the world might be teaching, gardening, cleaning, cooking, music, entrepreneurship, or simply doing a job with complete attentiveness and a desire to do your best.

Dedicated to Doing

Throughout time, many historical figures have escaped from this world of doing to simply be. Jesus retreated to the desert, the Buddha to the Bodhi Tree, and Thoreau to Walden. But if you look closely at the lives of those who fled society to *be*, you find something illuminating: They all came back to *do*.

Eventually most saints, mystics, philosophers, and sages returned to society. Even Thoreau, who scoffed at the need for friends, family, and social life during his two years and two months at Walden, came to this sobering conclusion, saying, "I left the woods for as good a reason as I went there. Perhaps it seemed to me that I had several more lives to live, and could not spare any more time for that one."[1]

What we learn from these luminaries is that being awake isn't enough. It's not enough to experience the fullness of each moment as a surfer in Maui, a monk in the Himalayas, or a yogi in India. Life isn't just about being. It isn't just about you and your connection to the present moment.

The world's enduring wisdom traditions tell us that a life well lived is also about what we *do* and the impact that we have on others. This is why all the great philosophers and prophets came back. They realized that waking up wasn't the end. It was the beginning. They realized that the essential task of living isn't to stop doing and start being. It's much bigger than that. It is to be *while* doing—to inspire and enhance the lives of those around us.

Informed by this critical distinction, the LIFE XT program stresses the importance of balancing these two experiences. If you delve too deeply into doing—if your whole life becomes consumed with meetings, work, and to-do lists—you may have a great impact on the world, but you miss out on the exquisite, everyday experience of being. You will also likely be far less productive and effective than you could be. If you go too deeply into being—if your life becomes all about *your* practice and *your* experience of the present moment—you may miss out on opportunities to contribute to the lives of others, to participate in the exquisite sweetness of intimate relationships, and to feel the profound satisfaction that comes with being full engaged in your work. The art of living is to skillfully find ways to balance being and doing.

PRACTICE 7: ENGAGEMENT

Dave and Sandra sit on opposite sides of the large meeting-room table, surrounded by ten other company managers. They are in the same room at the same meeting, but their experiences couldn't be more different.

Twenty minutes into the meeting, Dave starts to feel bored. He can't seem to get comfortable, alternately slumping in his chair and then straightening up. Every few minutes, he surreptitiously checks his phone for new email messages. He tracks the overall theme of the meeting but loses the details. He has little to contribute and soon starts to feel sleepy. Now he's counting down the minutes until the end of the meeting. How can it be only 10:39 a.m.? He feels like he has been here for hours. The voices of his coworkers drone on in the background while his attention focuses on a single thought: *When is this meeting finally going to end?*

Sandra sits tall in her chair on the other side of the table, alert yet relaxed in both body and mind. She listens carefully to the comments of others in the group and jumps at the opportunity to contribute to the conversation. She's not thinking about the time. She's focused on the task at hand.

Dave and Sandra are not only on opposite sides of the table; they sit on opposite sides of the spectrum of engagement.

Dave is living in a state of disengagement. Most of us have experienced this state at work, at a dinner party, or in a class. You feel exhausted, unproductive, and bored. You'd rather be anywhere else.

Sandra, by contrast, is living in a state of full engagement. You've probably experienced this state, too—in the exquisite feeling of finding yourself completely absorbed in a task or a moment. Time melts away. You feel energized and excited. Quantum leaps in productivity become possible, and you can effortlessly complete a huge volume of work in a matter of hours.

Given the choice, most of us would choose to be engaged. Yet in practice, our lives are often set up in such a way that the experience of full engagement is rare.

The Engagement practice is designed to help you become more fully aware of when you fall into disengagement. It provides tools that enable you to shift to a more fully engaged state, which can have life-changing implications. The state of full engagement leads to a greater sense of purpose, it transforms work into play, and it opens a space for more productive and creative output.

WHAT IT IS

You can distill much of the LIFE XT program down to a single axiom. In the words of William James, "My experience is what I agree to attend to."[1] When we allow the set point mind to run free, our attention wanders through worries, anxieties, and other negative states. When we learn to direct our attention, we create a different life experience.

Directing your full attention toward the task at hand—whatever it might be—gives you entrée into this state of full engagement. Mihaly Csikszentmihalyi was one of the first psychologists to research this experience. In his now-classic book *Flow*, he describes engagement—what he calls flow—as "the state in which people are so involved in an activity that nothing else seems to matter; the experience itself is so enjoyable that people will do it even at great cost, for the sheer sake of doing it."[2]

On its surface, engagement sounds a lot like presence, and they are in fact closely related. By definition, you can experience presence anytime, anywhere: lying on the beach, walking to your car, or sitting in traffic. It can be either passive or active. Engagement, on the other hand, is a purely active state that arises in specific conditions: when we use a skill we have developed to overcome some sort of challenge. In fact, the ideal conditions for engagement arise when, in Csikszentmihalyi's words, "both challenges and skills are high and equal to each other."[3]

Many top athletes, artists, and intellectuals describe this experience. Pelé, the iconic Brazilian soccer star, describes it like this: "I felt I could run all day without tiring, that I could dribble through any of their team or all of them, that I could almost pass through them physically."[4]

Musicians also experience this state. Buster Williams, the legendary jazz bassist, recalls that playing with Miles Davis led to this heightened state of engagement. "With Miles, it would get to the point where we followed the music rather than the music following us. We just followed the music wherever it wanted to go."[5]

These descriptions can make engagement sound mystical—like an otherworldly state. But you don't have to be a highly trained, acclaimed professional to experience engagement. It is a state of doing that everyone can access: on a challenging morning run, during an important PTA meeting, or while delivering a presentation at work. Csikszentmihalyi's research, for example, found that full-time caregivers were just as likely to experience this state as athletes and musicians. One mother described engagement happening when she worked with her child as her daughter was discovering something new. "Her reading is one thing that she's really into, and we read together. She reads to me, and I read to her, and that's a time when I sort of lose touch with the rest of the world. I'm totally absorbed in what I am doing."[6]

Cultivating this state of engagement requires integrating all of the other practices of LIFE XT. Engagement, after all, is the ultimate experience of being and doing. When you experience flow, you experience being—you are awake to the moment. Yet this experience arises in the midst of doing.

Let's try it right now with a seemingly easy task (one that you may recall from your childhood). It's a task that should be just challenging enough to take you into a state of engagement. Stand up and then pat your head with one hand while rubbing your belly in a circle with your other hand. If this is easy for you, add a more advanced move: Tap your left foot each time the hand that is patting your head reaches its highest point. See if you can do this for just thirty seconds.

Now check in again. Chances are that you were so focused on getting the movement right that the forces of the set point mind started to drop away. For thirty seconds your mind wandering probably faded into the background. This is a short taste of the experience of flow. It's the challenging yet enjoyable experience of becoming absorbed in the task at hand—an experience that can be difficult, even stressful, but it promotes wellbeing on all levels: mentally, emotionally, and physically.

The Engagement practice will give you the tools to begin developing the essential life skill of flow. You will start by building into your days a distraction-free time for fully engaged activity. We call this the Offline 30. You will then explore several other tools for maximizing your level of engagement: tips for identifying areas of flow and strategies for managing your energy while you work and using the moment-to-moment practice of Notice-Shift-Rewire to catch yourself in the midst of distraction and shift back to engaged work.

WHY IT WORKS

Ancient philosophy and modern psychology agree on this truth: Entering this fully engaged state is at the very core of happiness and wellbeing.

Some of the earliest references to the idea of engagement arise from the Taoist tradition of the East. The ancient Taoist scholar Chuang Tzu used the word *yu*—"wandering," "swimming," or "flowing"[7]—to describe this heightened state of doing.[8] "*Yu* was the proper way to live," Csikszentmihalyi explains, "without concern for external rewards, spontaneously, with total commitment."[9]

As a demonstration, Chuang Tzu tells the tale of a butcher experiencing flow while cutting up an ox. "The blade flashed and hissed" as he cut up the ox, writes Chuang Tzu, "its rhythm centered and ancient and never faltering."[10] The butcher says,

Way [engagement/flow] is all I care about, and Way goes beyond mere skill. When I first began cutting up oxen, I could see nothing but the ox. And now . . . I've stopped looking with my eyes . . . Keeping my skill constant and essential, I just slip the blade through, never touching ligament or tendon, let alone bone.[11]

What Chuang Tzu's butcher describes is engagement. It's the state that arises when being and doing come together.

The experience of engagement isn't just an Eastern phenomenon. During the Renaissance, the Italian philosopher Machiavelli experienced this ecstatic state while reading the great works of ancient philosophy and history each evening. In his words:

> *When evening comes, I return home and enter my study . . . I step inside the venerable courts of the ancients, where, solicitously received by them, I nourish myself on the food that* alone *is mine and for which I was born; where I am unashamed to converse with them and to question them about the motives for their actions, and they, out of their human kindness, answer me. And for four hours at a time, I feel no boredom, I forget all my troubles, I do not dread poverty, and I am not terrified by death. I absorb myself into them completely.*[12]

For Machiavelli, engagement erased the many distractions of the mind. It offered a rare opportunity to dive so deeply into the object of his focus—in this case reading—that everything else fell away. And Machiavelli's capacity for engagement was likely what enabled him to create some of the most influential works of political philosophy in Western history.

Ancient traditions point to the connection between flow and wellbeing. Yet it wasn't until the mid-1970s that psychologists like Csikszentmihalyi started to investigate the inner workings of this experience. Csikszentmihalyi interviewed thousands of artists, musicians, and athletes about their experiences of engagement. He found that during flow, a common cluster of experiences arises:

- The task is challenging and requires skill.
- You must concentrate.
- There are clear goals.
- You get immediate feedback.
- You experience a deep, effortless involvement.
- You experience a sense of control.

- Your sense of self vanishes.
- Time seems to stop.[13]

Csikszentmihalyi found the first of these qualities to be particularly important. Flow requires challenge. It can't happen while sitting on the couch watching TV or surfing the Internet. Instead, this state resides in the narrow gap between anxiety and boredom.[14]

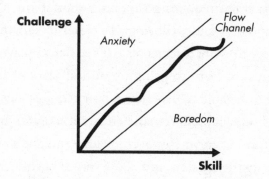

"Flow" concept by Mihaly Csikszentmihalyi. Drawn by Senia Maymin.

Sonja Lyubomirsky explains, "Whether you are rock climbing, performing surgery, doing your taxes, or driving on the freeway, if the challenges of the situation overwhelm your level of skill or expertise, you will feel anxious or frustrated ... If the activity is not challenging enough, you will become bored. Flow is a way of describing the experience that falls in just the right space between boredom and anxiety."[15]

This raises an important question. Given the many benefits of experiencing flow, why don't we challenge ourselves in ways that allow us to experience this state all the time? Why do we spend so much time swinging between boredom and anxiety?

As we have seen in the chapter on set point, the most basic answer is that we are attached to pleasure and resistant to pain. As humans, we are wired to pursue short-term pleasures. Our tendency is to take the shortest possible route to happiness—to find it in that extra bowl of ice cream or in hours spent watching television. These quick and easy pleasures give us immediate gratification, but they keep us from experiencing flow. Martin Seligman explains, "in the nightly choice between reading a good book and watching a sitcom on television, we often choose the latter—although surveys show that the average mood while watching sitcoms on television is mild depression."[16]

The challenge here is that entering the "flow channel" isn't always easy. It often requires postponing short-term pleasure for long-term happiness and wellbeing. It's easier to surf the Internet than it is to try to write a screenplay. It's easier to play a game on your phone than to learn to paint a beautiful work of art. Attaining the skills to be able to experience flow requires a considerable investment of time and effort—and frustration on the initial steep slope of the learning curve. But over the long run, the activities that allow you to experience flow also allow you to maximize your creative and productive potential. Flow not only makes us happier. It also makes us more successful at whatever we choose to do.

Csikszentmihalyi's research illuminates this connection between flow and wellbeing. In one study, his team had 250 high-flow and 250 low-flow teenagers keep a record of their mood at specific times throughout the day. When the team examined the responses, the low-flow teens spent the bulk of their time in a state of disengagement, hanging out at the mall or watching television. The high-flow teens, by contrast, were more likely to spend their time developing hobbies, academic interests, and athletic abilities.

How did these two groups score on measures of happiness? It turned out that the high-flow group outperformed the low-flow group on every measure of psychological wellbeing, except one. Seligman writes, "The exception is important: the high-flow kids think their low-flow peers are having more fun, and say they would rather be at the mall doing all those 'fun' things or watching television."[17] The only disadvantage of experiencing flow, in other words, was the feeling of missing out on short-term pleasures—pleasures that, in the end, fail to produce long-term happiness.

Two helpful conclusions can be drawn from this research. First, engagement cultivates happiness and wellbeing. The more we live in the state of flow, the more we grow and experience meaningful success. Second, flow doesn't always come naturally. We often have to resist the temptation of short-term pleasure to get there. When we do, we set the stage for this exquisite experience of total absorption in the task at hand.

HOW TO DEVELOP THIS SKILL

Habit 7: Engagement

How to do it: The LIFE XT Engagement practice is a simple ritual that you can build into each day. We call it the Offline 30. Each day, reserve thirty minutes or more for engaged and undistracted work (whatever pursuit you choose to call work). Turn off your phone, close your web browser and email, shut off the TV, even shut down your router if you have to. Do whatever you need to do to eliminate the countless digital distractions that call for your attention. This straightforward and effective practice will enhance wellbeing on all levels, helping you to become less distracted, more focused, productive, and inspired.

For more practical tips and strategies for building the habit of engagement, see the chapter "How to Practice Life Cross Training" at the end of the book.

Beyond the Offline 30:
Engagement in the Rest of Life

The Engagement practice is the first step toward living with a greater sense of flow. But for those who already have their own version of the Offline 30 or who are just interested in going deeper, here are a few additional tips for experiencing more flow in the midst of your everyday life.

Tip 1: Find Your Flow

For some lucky individuals, flow comes almost naturally. Mozart started playing concerts at age six. Picasso painted his first masterpiece at eight. People like Mozart and Picasso don't have to consciously train the skill of engagement. From early on, this experience of total absorption in the task at hand becomes a way of life.

For most of us, however, dropping into this state of flow requires a bit more practice and reflection. The first step is to identify activities that offer the potential for flow. You may already have a few activities in mind. But to help you identify other potential flow activities, consider the things you do, either at work or at home, that meet the following criteria:

1. *Challenge.* Remember that flow doesn't arise when things are easy. Quite the opposite. Flow arises when we push our skills and abilities to their very limit. What are the activities that challenge you?

2. *Enthusiasm.* Flow and lack of interest don't go well together. Passion is a prerequisite for this state. You have to enjoy what you are doing to be in a state of engagement. What are the things you love to do?

3. *Skill.* Flow requires a certain level of mastery. A beginning student learning to play her first song on the piano is less likely to experience flow than a concert pianist with twenty years of experience. You don't have to achieve complete mastery, but achieving a high level of skill is essential. What are your most highly developed or natural skills?

Write your answers to these three questions on a sheet of paper. See if you can identify three to five activities for each question.

Now look for any common themes in your responses. The activities at work or at home that showed up in two or three of these questions are good candidates for developing the experience of engagement. When you find something that combines challenge, enthusiasm, and skill, you have found your individual recipe for engagement. This is an activity you can begin to use as your portal into the experience of flow.

The final step is to think about the environment that will promote this experience. This is particularly important in your career. Each company and work environment promotes a distinctive kind of engagement. If you feel flow while writing alone on your computer, then a job in sales at a company with a sprawling open floor plan probably isn't the best fit. If you thrive on constant change and innovation, then working for a large international corporation might not suit you best.

If, however, you can find a way to match your flow activities with a work environment that allows you to develop these skills, you will not only experience more engagement but will find that you enjoy going to work each day, live with a deeper sense of purpose, and will likely be much more successful in your profession.

Tip 2: Live and Work in Flow

Once you have identified the activities that offer the potential for flow, the next step is to integrate this experience into your everyday life—to maximize the amount of time spent in this state. This requires optimizing the way you approach your life and your work. To build more flow experiences into our work lives, we must first understand the dynamics of physical and mental energy that produce this state.

Let's start with the problem. When it comes to work, we live in a culture that promotes an atmosphere of near-constant action—a frenetic state of being that makes it feel as if we're missing out if we are not constantly doing. Red Bull and other energy-boosting products have become a multibillion-dollar industry. The culture of the modern workplace makes matters worse. It is based on the socially reinforced ideal of continuous exertion—the more hours we can work, the tougher, stronger, more attractive, and more valuable we are. Even our rare moments of leisure time have become opportunities for constant doing. On Facebook, Instagram, and other social media outlets, we see a live stream of the doings of other people: vacations, achievements, and exciting events.

The problem is that our bodies and minds weren't designed to do this. Physiologist Martin Moore-Ede explains:

> *Our bodies were designed to hunt by day, sleep at night and never travel more than a few dozen miles from sunrise to sunset. Now we work and play at all hours, whisk off by jet to the far side of the globe, make life-or-death decisions or place orders on foreign stock exchanges in the wee hours of the morning . . . We are* machine-centered *in our thinking . . . rather than* human-centered—*focused on the optimization of human alertness and performance.*[18]

From this machine-centered view, it can seem like we ought to be able to live in a constant state of flow. We ought to be able to write emails for twelve hours at a time, schedule back-to-back-to-back business trips, and host elaborate dinner parties every night.

But we're not machines. We're human. And because of our biology and prehistoric roots, the experience of full engagement requires that we intersperse periods of intense focus with periods of recovery. It requires that we learn the art of what Jim Loehr and Tony Schwartz, authors of *The Power of Full Engagement*, call sprint and recover.

Loehr and Schwartz's big idea is that maximizing productivity and this experience of flow requires oscillation. "Full engagement," they write, "requires cultivating a dynamic balance between the expenditure of energy (stress) and the renewal of energy (recovery) in all dimensions [physical, emotional, mental, and spiritual]."[19]

We understand this concept when it comes to athletics. It would be crazy to train for a marathon by running a marathon each day. Instead, it is intuitively obvious that we are better served by running a variety of distances at a variety of speeds, mixing intense physical stress with rest and recovery.

The same principle holds for our mental and emotional energy. If we try to live up to this cultural ideal of continuous exertion and attempt to experience full engagement for hours on end without oscillation, we soon end up feeling distracted and disengaged. When, on the other hand, we learn to sprint and then recover—mix periods of intense focus with periods of recovery—we become more productive, creative, and fully engaged throughout the day.

The legendary golfer Jack Nicklaus, winner of eighteen major championships, insists that this insight was one of the keys to his success. In his words,

I was blessed with the ability to focus intensely on whatever I'm doing through most distraction and usually to the exclusion of whatever else might otherwise preoccupy me. Nevertheless, I can't concentrate on nothing but golf shots for the time it takes to play eighteen holes. I've developed a regimen that allows me to move from peaks of concentration into valleys of relaxation and back again as necessary.

My focus begins to sharpen as I walk onto the tee, then steadily intensifies as I complete the process of analysis and evaluation that produces a clear-cut strategy for every shot I play. It then peaks as I set up to the ball and execute the swing when, ideally, my mind picture of what I'm trying to do is both totally exclusionary and totally positive.

I descend into a valley as I leave the tee, either through casual conversation with a fellow competitor or by letting my mind dwell on whatever happens into it.[20]

Loehr and Schwartz call it sprint and recover. Nicklaus calls it peaks and valleys. The idea is the same: Optimal engagement comes from alternating between moments of intense focus and moments of rest and renewal. Whether it is physical fitness, writing a novel, or designing a new computer algorithm, when we learn to alternate between intense states of focus and brief moments of recovery, we create the ideal conditions for achieving peak performance in all aspects of life.

Tip 3: Use Notice-Shift-Rewire to Shift from Pleasure to Flow

Engagement can be exhilarating. Yet, as we now know, the state of flow also entails challenge. It often arises when we push ourselves to the very limit. Climbing a thousand-foot vertical face, writing the final pages of a novel, or perfecting a Mozart sonata—these activities can involve fear of failure, physical pain, and intense periods of stress. Engagement isn't all ease and flow.

This presents a problem. The biologically driven forces of the set point lead us to attach to pleasure and resist pain. And let's face it, the distractions of modern life—TV, smartphones, and social media—can be quite pleasurable, at least in the short term. Researchers have found, for example, that receiving a text or an email causes the brain to release a small amount of dopamine, the primary neurotransmitter involved in experiencing pleasure. This in turn leads to what psychologists call "dopamine loops"—seeking out more and more short-term rewards through continual stimulation.[21] It's exactly the same neurobiological process that drives all other forms of addiction. So we are not only surrounded by distractions but are also drawn to the short-term pleasure that they deliver. This is why we are more likely to prefer short-term pleasures like watching a reality TV show or surfing the Internet over other, more engaged activities.

But as we have seen throughout *Start Here*, the pathway to short-term pleasure isn't always the same as the path to happiness and wellbeing. The inner technology of Notice-Shift-Rewire gives us a tool for noticing the opportunities that arise in life for full engagement. By learning to Notice when we get seduced by pleasure-based shortcuts, we can shift our actions in ways that rewire our inherent biology and create a foundation for engagement-driven performance.

Step 1: Notice

The key to using Notice-Shift-Rewire for your Engagement practice is noticing when you unconsciously choose short-term pleasure over engaging in other, more meaningful endeavors. At work, notice when you start surfing the Internet or when you use sending emails as a way to avoid engaging fully in other work that may require more focus and effort. At home, notice each time you turn on the television or engage in other quick and easy pleasures.

These easy pleasures aren't bad. But they may stand in the way of experiencing more engagement and happiness in your life. Watching sports or reality TV programs, for example, isn't wrong. These activities work well as occasional periods of recovery after a fully engaged sprint. But if these shortcuts to happiness consistently stand in the way of reading a good book, having friends over, or taking up a hobby, then they may diminish your sense of aliveness over the long run.

Step 2: Shift

Noticing your attraction to short-term pleasure opens the possibility for change—for shifting from pleasure to flow.

Using the activities that you identified in the "Find Your Flow" section, shift your attention to those activities, skills, or tasks that require deep focus and engagement. It doesn't matter what you choose to do. You might write a letter to a friend, learn a musical instrument, start reading the complete works of Aristotle, or begin writing a report. What matters is that you are challenging yourself. Challenge, after all, is the gateway to full engagement.

Step 3: Rewire

Rewire through engaged doing. Be aware of what you are doing. Pay attention to what it feels like when you are fully engaged. Savor this state. Then forget about Notice-Shift-Rewire and allow yourself to become fully absorbed in the task at hand.

WHAT TO EXPECT

Just as you may have good days and bad days, you may have engaged days and distracted days. Yet turning the Offline 30 and the other tips for engagement into daily practices will increase the odds that the next time you settle down to write, play the piano, or cook a gourmet meal, you do so in a state of engagement—in a state where time falls away and you find yourself absorbed in the task at hand.

As you develop this habit, you will quickly encounter the challenge that we call the pleasure of distraction. As we have seen throughout *Start Here*, one of the most difficult obstacles to shifting our experience is the near-constant barrage of digital distractions we encounter each day—email, texts, Twitter, the Internet, and phone calls. These distractions bring us a seductive sense of pleasure and yet also stand in the way of flow.

Overcoming this urge toward distraction will likely be your primary challenge in building the habit of engagement. You will feel this most acutely during the initial stage of habit formation. It may take serious will and discipline to resist this pleasurable pull. As you dive into engaged work, you may feel drawn to your browser, phone, or email program. Notice the urge, witness the sensations and thoughts that arise along with it, and then shift your attention back to the task at hand. Rewire by staying with it.

With time and consistent practice, the experience of flow will become increasingly commonplace in your life. As this new habit takes hold, the first thing you will notice is a dramatic increase in your overall productivity at work and in life. Full engagement and intense focus allow you to do more in less time. You may also notice that you become increasingly confident and skilled in your work. You may begin to feel that there is no task you can't tackle. Previously daunting jobs will start to feel effortless as you approach them with focus and attention. People in your life may also start to notice these changes and turn to you for advice, support, and friendship. These changes come as you shift from distraction to flow.

At its core, engagement is the ultimate experience of LIFE XT in practice. It's the practice that enables you to begin to integrate being—drawing your attention to this moment—with doing: having an impact on the world through your work.

You will experience all of the benefits of LIFE XT in this one practice. Engagement reduces mind wandering, which is correlated to unhappiness. Engagement trains the skill of attention. Engagement allows us to choose where we place our thoughts and enables us to achieve a state of peak performance in all areas of our lives.

PRACTICE 8: RELATIONSHIPS

When it comes to illustrating the power of relationships, the life of Christopher McCandless serves as a cautionary tale.

Christopher was raised in an upper-middle-class family. He was an accomplished athlete and an avid hiker who loved exploring the outdoors. A star student, he graduated with honors from Emory University. But that's where his life took an unexpected and fateful turn.

Christopher wasn't enticed by the trappings of a normal life—a job, a life in the suburbs with a wife and kids. A young man driven by a mix of angst and alienation and the romance of testing himself against nature, he wanted to escape from relationships and social connections and venture out into the world alone.

Soon after commencement day at Emory, Christopher vanished. He donated his $20,000 savings to Oxfam International and left his comfortable life behind. For the next two years, he traveled the country using the name Alexander Supertramp.

Throughout his travels, Christopher preached a gospel of rugged individualism and isolation to those he met. He held the view that happiness arises not from human relationships, but from living in nature, alone.

An intense desire to find happiness outside the social world inspired his most daring adventure. In early April 1992, he ventured alone into the last frontier of the Alaskan wilderness. Jon Krakauer, who chronicled McCandless's life in the book *Into the Wild*, re-counts that Christopher left behind his map, "his watch, his comb, and all his money, which amounted to 85 cents."[1] All he had was a small thirty-pound backpack full of basic supplies.

For the first few weeks, Christopher felt exhilarated. He found a dilapidated bus that he turned into a makeshift cabin. He spent his days reading, reflecting, hunting for game, and living off the land.

But soon the challenge of surviving without the comforts of society started to get real. He struggled to find game. He started losing weight. Most surprising, he started to crave the one thing he had worked so hard to escape: relationships.

His journal, later found in the bus, chronicled his thoughts. On July 2, after reading Tolstoy's "Family Happiness," Christopher had a profound change of heart. He wrote about his own desire for happiness through the pursuit of being useful to others and the possibility of having his own family. His extreme experiment in social isolation led Christopher to the realization that "the only certain happiness in life is to live for others."[2]

Two days later, Christopher packed his bag and headed back for civilization, back to the world of family, friends, and associates. As you may already know from the book or the film based on it, Christopher's story ended tragically. To return to civilization, he had to cross the Teklanika River, which just two months earlier had still been frozen and thus easy to cross. Now it was a rushing river flooded with snowmelt—seventy-five feet wide and impassable. Unable to cross the Teklanika, Christopher retreated back into the wilderness.

Eventually he died of starvation. It's easy to write off Christopher as an idealistic social recluse who learned the hard way just how difficult it is to survive outside of society. But his story is also a lesson in the essential nature of relationships. Christopher pushed the solitary life to its very limit, one man against the world. In the end, he discovered that the key to happiness and even survival isn't just inner clarity, living in the present moment, or self-exploration. Happiness and wellbeing also arise from deep and satisfying relationships with the people we love.

The Relationships practice is based on the idea that you don't have to venture into the Alaskan wilderness to understand the value of relationships and begin nurturing them. Building relationships is an essential life skill that you can practice each day, a practice that can radically enhance your physical and emotional wellbeing.

WHAT IT IS

It is easy to think LIFE XT is a program for development of the self. When you inquire, meditate, or move, after all, the practice is about shifting *your* happiness set point.

The Do stage marks a pivotal point of transition, a shift from being in the moment to contributing to the world through deep engagement, strong relationships, and service to others. The Relationships practice is of particular importance. At the core of this practice is a key idea: Relationships and wellbeing go hand in hand. In fact, they work together to create a kind of upward spiral of a life well lived. Healthy relationships sow the seeds of optimal wellbeing. They strengthen your immune system, allow you to live longer, and make you more resilient to stress. Yet the opposite is also true: Wellbeing strengthens our relationships. Those who feel healthy, happy, and content in their lives make betters friends, co-workers, lovers, and life partners.

While almost everyone already has important relationships, the

Relationships practice gives you a new way to think about investing in them. Many of us are poor decision makers when it comes to optimizing wellbeing. We tend to think that success in the form of money, status, and professional advancement leads to wellbeing. Yet these very pursuits can often have the opposite effect, taking time away from our most cherished connections.

The Relationships practice gives you an evidence-based argument that when it comes to wellbeing, investing in relationships delivers better results. The practice involves building a simple ritual into each week—the Weekly Connection. It might be a date night with your spouse, a walk with a friend, or an outing to an amusement park with your child. It's a weekly opportunity to tune out the many distractions of modern life and tune in to the people you love. In addition to this weekly ritual, you will further develop your ability to show up fully in your relationships—to be fully present with the people in your life.

WHY IT WORKS

The texts of ancient wisdom traditions, philosophical treatises, and the fMRI studies of modern neuroscience all point to relationships as an essential ingredient in living a good life. Enduring wisdom teaches that healthy relationships offer a direct pathway to thriving in all areas of life. Modern science tells us that feeling connected to others changes our behavior in many surprising ways that improve our health and overall wellbeing such as improved sleep, better eating habits, and a longer life.

The theme of relationships runs throughout many ancient texts. And yet the most influential discussion of relationships in the West arises from the writings of Aristotle.

In his classic text *The Nicomachean Ethics*, Aristotle devotes two of the final chapters to the topic of relationships. His big idea: Life wouldn't be worth living without relationships. "Nobody," he writes, "would choose to live without friends even if he had all the other good things."[3]

To say that Aristotle's reflections in this area have been influential is an understatement. His work on relationships (he uses the Greek word for friendship, *philia*) has shaped the thinking of just about every serious Western philosopher and spiritual thinker.[4]

Aristotle focuses on friendship. Friendship, he tells us, "is not only a necessary thing but a splendid one."[5] Aristotle wanted to understand what distinguishes various types of friendships. As we all know, not all friendships are created equal. Some inspire us to thrive, while others keep us locked in drama. New technologies make categorizing friendships even more complicated. Many of us have hundreds or even thousands of "friends" on Facebook, LinkedIn, Instagram, and other social networking sites.

So how do you distinguish between your deepest friendships and the random person who sent you a "friend" request after a two-minute conversation? Aristotle's answer was to divide friendships into three categories: friendships based on utility, friendships based on pleasure, and perfect friendships.

Friendships based on utility arise when friends "take pleasure in each other's company only in so far as they have hopes of advantage from it."[6] These friendships are transactional. They're the kinds of bonds that we make when we're expanding our circle of influence to gain some professional advantage or social convenience. These relationships aren't bad. In fact, they are often necessary. But they are the relational equivalent of negotiating for a lower price at your local car dealership. You might be friendly with one another and even like each other. But at the end of the day, these relationships operate on the principle of *I get mine and you get yours.* The moment the exchange of utility breaks down, the friendship is over.

Pause for a moment. Think about the people in your life. Who in your life fits the description of friendships of utility?

Aristotle's second category—friendships based purely on pleasure—can arise in any number of ways. They can be sexual (Aristotle tells us that many of these relationships have an "erotic" side to them); but they can also be based on other forms of pleasure. You might be friends with someone because he or she makes you laugh, has an exceptional fashion sense, or has fascinating stories to tell. The motto of these friendships might be something like *We're friends—so long as it feel good.*

Pause again. Think again about past or present relationships in your life. How many of your relationships are based primarily on some form of pleasure?

For Aristotle, the first two forms of friendship are incomplete and ultimately unsatisfying. Real friendship isn't about what you get or how much pleasure you experience. Real friendship, what Aristotle calls perfect friendship, is about loving others for their own sake. And it is through loving others for their own sake that we experience increased wellbeing and happiness.

Jill Bolte Taylor, author of *My Stroke of Insight,* describes feeling this deep experience of love. As she lay in her hospital bed in the ICU just after suffering a massive stroke, her mother entered the room for the first time. Because her left hemisphere had been severely damaged by the stroke, Taylor had no concept of "mother" at the time. But that didn't interfere with the experience of love. In her words, her mother

> *lifted my sheet and proceeded to crawl into bed with me. She immediately wrapped me up in her arms and I melted into the familiarity*

of her snuggle. It was an amazing moment in my life. Somehow she understood that I was no longer her Harvard doctor daughter, but instead I was now her infant again . . . Having been born to my mother was truly my first and greatest blessing. Being born to her a second time has been my greatest fortune.[7]

Pause one last time. Think about the relationships in your life (friends, family, children, parents) where you love others for their own sake. How many of your relationships fall into this category?

Your answers to these questions may reveal some interesting insights. If the bulk of your time is devoted to relationships based on utility and pleasure, consider ways to cultivate the relationships where you love others for their own sake. At its core, this is an exercise in prioritization and time management. Make an extra effort to set aside time for your authentic relationships and think carefully about whether to say yes to social engagements based purely on utility and pleasure. Following this important prescription will free up more time in your schedule and deepen your relationships.

This raises a question: *How do we cultivate more of these authentic, "perfect" relationships?* Aristotle's answer harkens back to the Compassion practice: *love.* If you want real friends and lasting relationships, you must love the people in your life. Even more important, you must be more interested in "giving than in receiving affection."[8] Others benefit from the support and love that we offer, but so do we. "In its extreme form," says Aristotle, "friendship approximates to self-love."[9] In another passage, he explains that the "feelings that we have towards our neighbors . . . seem to be derived from our feelings towards ourselves."[10]

Here we return to the idea that relationships work like a mirror: We tend to get back what we put out. This means that the more we blame, criticize, and resent those closest to us, the more we begin to feel bad about ourselves. We live in a culture that often rein-forces this pattern. TV shows, blogs, and social media sites thrive on judgment, criticism, and shaming. This pattern also shows up in ordinary life: from time to time all of us slip into "talk trash" (gossip) about others. Aristotle's insight reveals that these actions are ultimately self-destructive. The more we indulge this habit, the more we begin to subconsciously subject ourselves to this very same barrage of judgment, blame, and criticism. That's the dark side of the mirror you've probably experienced more than once.

But we can also choose to flip that mirror: The more love and affection we send out to others in our lives, the more we get back. Aristotle explains, "In loving a friend [we] are loving [our] own good."[11] This is a powerful idea. It means that if you want more love, connection, and support from others, change starts with you. By training your ability to put out more love, more presence, and more compassion, you not only improve the chances that others will mirror back these qualities but also begin to feel more love for yourself. This insight from Aristotle will be helpful to carry with you as you begin the practice of strengthening your relationships.

Aristotle understood at an intuitive level the profound value of relationships. Over the last thirty years, a growing body of research in the field of neuroscience has begun to validate that intuition. John Cacioppo, the author of *Loneliness: Human Nature and the Need for Social Connection*,[12] has shown in his research that human interaction, or lack thereof, leads to significant alterations in brain functioning—for better and for worse.

It turns out that social disconnection has the effect of impairing executive functioning, the capacity of the brain to control thoughts and impulses. When we suffer from a lack of healthy relationships, we become more impulsive, more anxious, and less emotionally resilient. These emotional consequences spill over into the physical realm. Loneliness, says Cacioppo, leads to the kinds of impulsive behaviors that, while pleasurable, damage our physical health: eating fatty and sugary foods, drinking in excess, abusing drugs, and not exercising.

Consider whether this is true in your life. When you feel lonely or feel that you lack connection in your life, how does your behavior change? Do you sleep as well? Do you eat differently?

An experiment conducted by Roy Baumeister offers a shocking illustration of how our behavior changes under these conditions. Baumeister and his research team had a group of volunteer participants mingle with one another. Their task was to find a group of people whom they trusted and respected. Rather than forming groups on the spot, however, participants gave researchers the names of the two people they most wanted to work with following the event.

Baumeister's team then called the participants back for a follow-up session. In this session, researchers portrayed half of the participants as outcasts. They were told bluntly that nobody chose them. "That's fine," they were told, "you can just go ahead and complete the next part of the task alone."[13] Researchers portrayed the other half as group favorites. They were told that *everyone* in the room wanted to work with them, but because it was too difficult to assign them to a small group, they would do the task by themselves.[14]

Then researchers brought in a bowl of thirty-five chocolate chip cookies. All the subjects were told they would be participating in a "taste test." They were told they could eat as many cookies as they needed to offer a sound assessment of their flavor.

What happened next? The group "favorites"—those who

felt loved and accepted—ate four or five cookies on average. The "outcasts"—those who felt the sting of rejection—ate twice as many cookies. This is clear evidence that when we feel lonely, rejected, or isolated from others, we become more prone to unhealthy behaviors.

The problem is not so much that loneliness itself makes you unhealthy. It's that the emotions associated with being alone tend to compromise our executive functioning, which in turn sets off a cascade of damaging biological consequences.[15] In fact, Cacioppo's research points to a direct biological link between loneliness and diminished wellbeing. In addition to compromising executive functioning, Cacioppo's team has also found that feeling alone is associated with increased levels of stress hormones: Loneliness the day before, they concluded, is directly correlated with an increase in cortisol levels the next morning.[16] By placing additional stress on the mind and body, feeling lonely has a whole host of other negative effects: increased inflammation, reduced immunity, and increased rates of mortality.[17]

So for those of us interested in living a happier life, the evidence shows that relationships play a pivotal role in cultivating wellbeing. In fact, the evidence points to a mutually reinforcing connection between relationships and happiness. Sonja Lyubomirsky observes, "This means that romantic partners and friends make people happy, but it also means that happy people are more likely to acquire lovers and friends."[18]

This is the "upward spiral" of relationships: Strengthening our relationships makes us happier, and being happier strengthens our relationships.

HOW TO DEVELOP THIS SKILL

Before we outline the Relationships practice, it's important to point out a deep paradox that many people encounter in their closest relationships. In a world of constant busyness, it's easy for many of us to invest in "productive" activities at the expense of relationships. We're driven by what psychologists call the *hedonic treadmill*—by the idea that if we work more, we will make more (either now or later), which will, in the end, make us and our families happy. Driven by this mostly unconscious belief, many of us end up placing work ahead of spending quality time with the people we love most.

The problem is, this seductive belief is just plain wrong. Studies show that the more we make, the more we begin to crave new, unattainable things. One such study examined perceptions of wealth over a thirty-five-year period. Researchers found that each increase in wealth corresponded to an increase in desire. Lyubomirsky explains, "the estimate for 'get along' income increased almost exactly to the same degree as did actual income, suggesting that the more you have, the more you think you 'need.'"[19]

It's important to consider just how absurd this is. Without thinking about it, many of us instinctively prioritize emails, meetings, and phone calls over being present with our spouses, playing soccer with our children, or helping our neighbor who just had back surgery.

We think this trade-off will somehow make us happy. But the science is clear: It won't.

There is a better way to think about investing time. What we know from ancient wisdom and modern science is that relationships are resistant to this phenomenon of hedonic adaptation. Investing in our kids, our marriages, or our friendships actually makes us happier and healthier. This isn't to say that you should quit your job and invest every waking moment in relationships. But if you notice yourself consistently prioritizing work over the people you love, you would be well served to focus more of your attention on the Relationships practice.

Habit 8: Relationships

How to do it: The LIFE XT Relationships practice involves building a ritual into your everyday life—the Weekly Connection. Most of us already spend significant amounts of time in the physical presence of people we love. But simply being *with* them isn't the same as being *connected to* the people we love. Research in psychology, for example, shows that it's the quality, not the quantity, of time spent with children that has the most profound effect on behavioral, emotional, and academic outcomes.[20] The Weekly Connection is your invitation to break out of the ordinary patterns of busyness and distraction. The practice is simple: Schedule one time each week to experience quality time with someone you love. For more practical tips and strategies for building the habit of relationships, see the chapter "How to Practice Life Cross Training" at the end of the book.

Beyond the Weekly Connection: Improving Relationships in the Rest of Life

We highly recommend making time for the people you love by weaving the Weekly Connection into your everyday life. But you can also improve your relationships by just being more present when you're in the company of your friends, spouse, or children—

even if you are just driving your kids to school or rushing through breakfast before work.

The key is to Notice-Shift-Rewire your attention. You don't have to be on a romantic date or a Saturday-morning excursion to the local zoo to feel connected. You just have to shift your attention from mind wandering and distraction to being present. In fact, this shift often becomes contagious. Your spouse, kids, friends, and family will feel the difference. Your shift to presence will open a space for them to feel more alive, supported, and loved. Of course, the reverse is also true. Your distraction is also contagious. It will make those around you feel more distant and uneasy.

Step 1: Notice

As we have seen, awareness and noticing is always the first step. It's easy to fall into bad habits, easy to distract yourself with the latest celebrity gossip or stock-market update in the presence of your loved ones. Noticing gives you a choice. Next time you reach for the remote while sitting next to your partner, notice. Next time you pull out your phone while your child is playing at the park, notice. Next time you lose yourself in a sea of worries while walking with a good friend, notice.

By training the skill of noticing, you open a space for showing up in a different, more present way in your relationships.

Step 2: Shift

The way to shift in this practice is by drawing your attention toward the present moment. It's the practice you worked on at the beginning of the Being section. In relationships, however, you are shifting toward a particular kind of presence. It's less about focusing inside, on your breath, and more about focusing your attention outward, on the person in front of you.

Step 3: Rewire

As you shift into a more present and available state, take a moment to savor and enjoy this new perspective. This shift will encode a new experience into your brain and nervous system. It will help build new superhighways of habit, turning the skill of showing up for your friends and family into a new way of doing. Try it today and see how you feel.

WHAT TO EXPECT

Aristotle offers a helpful first step for improving your relationships: Make sure that you are investing in the right relationships. You don't have to end all your friendships based on utility or pleasure. But for the purposes of this practice, we encourage you to focus your attention on building the deeper, more authentic connections in your life: those whom you love for their own sake.

The second step is to begin building this ritual into each week. For most of us, this requires addressing an uncomfortable reality: Life is busy. Whether you are a corporate executive or a stay-at-home parent, your days are likely filled with things to do. The primary challenge that stands in the way of building the Weekly Connection habit isn't a lack of love or affection for the people in your life; it's often a lack of advance planning and prioritization. To help you overcome this challenge, here are a couple of strategies that have worked well for us and participants in LIFE XT:

- *Schedule it on your calendar.* At the beginning of each month, take a few minutes to plan weekly opportunities for connection. Schedule time with the important people in your life.

Plan a couple of fun outings for your kids. Organize a hike with a friend.

- *Prioritize these dates.* Setting up these times for connection is relatively easy. Remembering to do it often isn't. It can be helpful to treat these appointments as the most important meetings in your week.

This logistical challenge sounds so obvious that you might be temped to skip over it. Yet it is one of the most difficult obstacles standing in the way of building deeper connections with loved ones.

The final and most important step is to fully show up during these times of connection. Especially when it comes to spending time with the people closest to us, it can be easy to slip into bad habits. When you are playing checkers with your child, it might be hard to ignore the sound of an incoming text. When you are having coffee with a friend, you might become distracted by that email you forgot to send before you left the office.

Scheduling is essential. But this more intangible skill of showing up for the people you love most is even more important. The good news is that you already have the recipe for this kind of quality, engaged time. It is something you have been developing throughout the course of LIFE XT. The key is to begin using time spent with friends and family as an opportunity to be in a state of presence, gratitude, and compassion. Relationships, it turns out, are the perfect training ground for refining your ability to Notice-Shift-Rewire.

So next time you are with your child, use this time as your cue to shift to presence. Really be there. Catch yourself when your mind wanders. Take note of the weather, the feeling of the breeze against your skin, and the sound of your child's laugh.

Next time you spend time with someone important in your life, use this as your cue to shift to gratitude. Tell this person what it is that you appreciate most about him or her. Remind yourself how lucky you are to have someone so amazing in your life.

Next time you see your extended family, use this as a cue to shift to compassion. Instead of focusing on their quirks and irritating qualities, redirect your attention to empathy and love. Feel what it might be like to walk in their shoes for a day. Be kind, gentle, and open.

This is the deepest form of LIFE XT practice—when habits like presence, relationships, and compassion become integrated into the everyday flow of life. And it's when you begin to experience the most profound physical and mental benefits of having close connections in your life: more affection, less conflict, and more of the exquisite experience of love.

PRACTICE 9: CONTRIBUTION

Imagine having your life turned upside down by a twitch in your pinkie finger.

That's exactly what happened to Michael J. Fox on a November morning in 1990. At the time, Fox was a twenty-nine-year-old superstar. Through his breakout roles in *Family Ties* and the Back to the Future trilogy, he had become one of America's most beloved celebrities. Fox had it all: fame, money, and the lavish life of a Hollywood star.

But when he woke up that morning, he received a message from his left hand that would change everything. In his words, "It wasn't a fax, telegram, memo, or the usual sort of missive bringing disturbing news. In fact, my hand held nothing at all. The trembling was the message."[1]

Fox wouldn't know the full meaning of that morning message for another year. But in time he learned that his life would never be the same. Doctors diagnosed Fox—just thirty years old—with Parkinson's disease, a degenerative neurological condition with no known cure.

The most remarkable thing about Fox's story is what happened next. He knew that he stood at the intersection of two paths. One path would be to, as he puts it, "adopt a siege mentality"—to become a victim of his situation and give up on life. The other path would be to "embark upon a journey"—to use this "neurological catastrophe" to find meaning and purpose in life.[2]

Fox chose the second path. His focus shifted from movies, television shows, and fame to finding a cure for the illness that plagued him and millions of others. He soon became a much-needed celebrity advocate for people living with Parkinson's and created the Michael J. Fox Foundation, which has raised $450 million to help find a cure for the disease.

Fox's little finger and the underlying neurological condition that made it twitch that day woke him up to a new way of looking at life. It led to what Fox calls an "apparent perversity" in the way he thinks of his life. As he explains, "If you were to rush into this room right now and announce that you had struck a deal . . . in which the ten years since my diagnosis could be magically taken away, traded in for ten more years as the person I was before—I would, without a moment's hesitation, tell you to take a hike."[3]

Fox had it all in his old life and, without Parkinson's, his success would have surely continued. But he describes his old life as resting on a flimsy foundation—on what he describes as a "sheltered, narrow existence fueled by fear and made livable by insulation, isolation, and self-indulgence."[4]

Before Parkinson's, Fox had money, fame, a family, and seemingly perfect health. But he was missing something deeper. His life lacked what he would soon find through his heartbreaking diagnosis: meaning, purpose, and the sense of deep contribution to the world.

The Contribution practice is based on the idea that you don't have to undergo a life-altering diagnosis to live with more meaning and purpose. We can all engage in this deep sense of meaning by developing our capacity to contribute.

WHAT IT IS

Contribution is closely and wonderfully related to the Be Stage Practice of Compassion. Where Compassion is a state of being, the inner experience of extending empathy and love to all beings, including yourself, Contribution is compassion externalized, the active expression of compassion. Acts of contribution allow us to *be* and *do*—to merge the inner experience of loving-kindness with outwardly focused acts of generosity toward others.

The act of contribution takes many different forms. You might donate your time at a local senior center. You might set aside a certain amount of money each year for charitable giving. Or you might engage in small random acts of kindness: giving up your seat on a crowded bus or helping the person in front of you on an airplane hoist a carry-on into the overhead bin.

Each day we experience countless opportunities to contribute to the lives of others. But in the midst of our ordinary mind wandering, we often miss these moments. It's easy to get so absorbed in thoughts about the trip you're planning or the argument you had last night that you become blind to these possibilities. The goal of the Contribution practice is to create a habit of noticing these everyday opportunities, shifting toward actions that contribute to the lives of those around us, and then rewiring by savoring the richness of the feeling that almost always accompanies the act.

Matthew, a thirty-three-year-old financial consultant in New York City, tells this story:

> *I manage people's money for a living, and I've always been uncomfortable with homeless people asking me for money—to the point where I would often cross the street to avoid them. But after a while*

I found that was just making me more aware of my own awkwardness around them, and of the change that was jingling in my pocket. I could afford to give someone a dollar or even five dollars, let alone a quarter. So one day on the way to work, I went out with the idea of giving some change to every panhandler I saw, just to see what would happen. I was taken completely by surprise by how good it made me feel. I noticed that I felt relieved, too—I think all that holding back was weighing on my spirit. The really weird thing was that I started being more open to helping in other ways—even holding the door for someone instead of rushing through it myself felt good. When I called my mom and asked if she needed me to bring her anything when I came to visit, she asked me if I was feeling okay.

Matthew's story offers an important reminder—your contribution doesn't have to involve large sums of money or traveling to a foreign land to help people. In fact, the final practice of Contribution will help you build such random acts of kindness into your everyday life. Even the subtlest actions—buying a homeless person a sandwich, helping a relative craft a résumé, or shoveling the snow off your neighbor's sidewalk—can have a profound impact on the lives of those around you. Try it today. Do one everyday act of kindness. Help your spouse, your coworker, your child, or a random person at the store. Notice the shift that you experience.

Like the Relationships practice, these random acts of kindness have a two-way effect. They improve the lives of those around us. And yet they also have a profound effect on our own wellbeing. Acts of contribution lead to increased optimism, enhanced immunity, and a neurological shift that scientists call the *helper's high.*

WHY IT WORKS

Throughout *Start Here*, we have navigated delicately around the subject of religion. Religious traditions hold profound insights for living a better life. LIFE XT seeks to offer a program with no single moral or religious foundation—a program that can be used by anyone, regardless of faith tradition. The concept of Contribution, however, is one area where all the major religions align around the same powerful idea: Giving of yourself is good.

In Judaism, we are told that "all men are responsible for one another" and that "he who prays for his fellow man, while he himself has the same need, will be answered first."[5] The Christian tradition echoes this theme, advising that "it is more blessed to give than to receive."[6] These traditions teach an important lesson: When it comes to contribution, even small everyday acts of kindness can change the lives of others. While it may be only a small amount of money for you, for someone else, it could be the exact amount that they need to buy their only meal of the day.

The Quran expands on this notion:

> *Each person's every joint must perform a charity every day the sun comes up: to act justly between two people is a charity; to help a man with his mount, lifting him onto it or hoisting up his belongings onto it, is a charity; a good word is a charity; every step you take to prayers is a charity; and removing a harmful thing from the road is a charity.*[7]

The point here is that every moment offers the possibility for charity and contribution. Generosity can be as easy as "removing a harmful thing from the road."

And yet the traditions also emphasize that giving by itself isn't sufficient. Motivation also plays a key role. Contribution isn't just about your actions. It's also about your motives—that is, acting for the sake of others, not yourself. The Hindu tradition advises, "Giving simply because it is right to give, without thought of return, at a proper time, in proper circumstances, and to a worthy person, is enlightened giving. Giving with regrets or in the expectation of receiving some favor or of getting something in return, is selfish giving."[8]

The point here isn't just theoretical. Proper intention is essential to the way you practice contribution. As you weave this practice into your day-to-day life, see if you can realize this art of enlightened giving. Contribute, not so you can get something in return, but for the sake of helping others. As Mother Teresa put it, "It's not how much we give but how much love we put into giving."

Over the last thirty years, researchers have amassed an overwhelming body of empirical evidence showing that the act of contributing to others—while working, volunteering, donating money, or even thinking about doing good—provides powerful physiological and neurological benefits.

David McClelland, a behavioral psychologist at Harvard, conducted one of the earliest studies in this area, revealing that simply *thinking* about contributing to the lives of others enhances our immune system. McClelland presented subjects with a short film about Mother Teresa's work with orphans in Calcutta. He then observed what came to be known as the Mother Teresa Effect: By watching the inspired example of someone like Mother Teresa contributing to the world, subjects showed significant and lasting increases in immunity.[9]

Subsequent studies have confirmed the powerful effect of

contribution. Studies of cardiac patients[10] and those with multiple sclerosis[11] show that when these people spend time supporting other patients their levels of depression decline, and they tend to live longer.[12]

The benefits of contribution also arise in the brain. Recent neurological imaging studies by Jorge Moll show that contribution generates a helper's high, which can be observed in the brain. In one study, researchers examined the effects of having subjects make a donation to a charity. This task resulted in the activation of the mesolimbic pathway—a primitive part of the brain that enables us to experience the dopamine-mediated pleasure that arises from eating and sex.[13]

This evidence helps explain why psychologists see contribution as such an essential gateway to cultivating meaning and purpose in our lives. In Martin Seligman's influential work *Flourish*, he identifies contribution as a central source of meaning in life: "The Meaningful Life consists in belonging to and serving something that you believe is bigger than the self, and humanity creates all the positive institutions to allow this: religion, political party, being green, the Boy Scouts, or the family."[14]

The research is clear: When we contribute to the lives of others, we experience enhanced physical health and overall wellbeing. Yet this is only a small part of why we advocate turning contribution into a habit. As we are reminded by the ancient wisdom traditions, giving of ourselves to the world is an activity that is worth doing for its own sake. True, you will feel happier and experience increases in immunity. But the real reason to contribute is that you will end up touching the lives of others. And for a just a moment, imagine what the world would be like if we all embraced this philosophy with equal vigor.

HOW TO DEVELOP THIS SKILL

Contribution is the ultimate win-win. Our everyday acts of kindness improve the lives of others while also enhancing our own well-being. Why, then, are they often so difficult to do? Why do many of us go through the day rarely, if ever, placing our attention on contributing to the lives of others?

A 1973 study conducted at the Princeton Theological Seminary helps shed light on the answer. In this now-classic experiment, John Darley and Daniel Batson divided Princeton seminary students into two groups. One group was told to deliver a sermon on the parable of the Good Samaritan (a timeless story of contribution). The other was told to deliver a talk about jobs for seminar students. They also added one other condition: Some students were told they had plenty of time, while others were told they needed to rush to the other building to deliver their talk.

This is where the experiment becomes interesting. On their way to the other building, participants encountered a man who was coughing, slumped over in pain, and clearly in need of help.

So here's the question: Which students stopped and which students kept on walking? The results showed that focusing on contribution mattered: 53 percent of the students tasked with talking about helping others stopped, while only 29 percent of the students delivering a talk on jobs stopped.

The most powerful factor, however, was whether or not students were in a rush. Only 10 percent of the students in a hurry stopped, compared to 63 percent of those who had plenty of time.[15]

For those of us who race through our days focused on our never-ending task list, this study has some uncomfortable implications. We all know that contribution is good for us and good for the world. Yet this study reveals that we pass up on the countless opportunities to contribute that arise each day, partially because our attention is elsewhere but also because we are in such a rush. For all of us, this study is a good reminder to make good on our intention to help others by slowing down and noticing when we can be of service to others.

Habit 9: Contribution

How to do it: This final LIFE XT practice will help you turn contribution into a regular routine. We call this performing everyday acts of kindness. The goal is to make these acts of service a weekly or even daily ritual. You don't need to donate millions or save someone's life for your act to count. A kind act that improves the life of a fellow being is all that is required. The field of possibilities is limitless. You could pick up a piece of trash off the sidewalk. You could pay the toll for the driver behind you. You could allow a rushed traveler to move ahead of you in an airport security line. As we will see, the real challenge lies in training your ability to notice—to become more aware of the opportunities for contribution that arise in almost every moment. For more practical tips and strategies for building the habit of contribution, see the chapter "How to Practice Life Cross Training" at the end of the book.

Performing Everyday Acts of Kindness

The most rewarding forms of contribution are often unplanned and improvisational. They arise in the moment: when you pass a motorist whose car just broke down or spot a child searching for his mother in a department store. The inner technology of Notice-Shift-Rewire is the perfect skill to help you become more alert and awake to these possibilities.

Step 1: Notice

The first step is to Notice—to become aware of the almost limitless opportunities to contribute. Consider a quick trip to the grocery store. You pull into the parking lot and notice a prime spot open in the front row. Do you dart into the spot or let the driver in the other lane take it? When you enter the store, you notice a woman in the produce aisle just tipped over a container of blueberries. Do you walk past as you continue shopping or stop to help her pick them up? At the checkout counter, you notice that the person behind you has only two items while you have a full cart. Do you let them ahead of you, or do you stick to your place in line? It's certainly not wrong to pass up these opportunities. In fact, we do just that every day—that's why small everyday acts of kindness can be so powerful. So as you go throughout your day-to-day life—as you ride the elevator in your office building, shop, dine out, drive, and talk with others—notice all the ways you could make someone else's day just a little bit better.

Step 2: Shift

At first, remembering to notice opportunities to contribute is the hard part. Shifting is much easier. It happens almost automatically when you make the choice to act in ways that improve the well-being of others. If you notice that you rarely contribute to charity, shifting is the act of writing that first check. If you notice that you tend to race ahead of other people so that you can get a better spot on the wait list at a busy restaurant, shifting is the act of slowing down and letting the people already ahead of you go first.

Step 3: Rewire

Notice-Shift-Rewire helps you remember to savor. Take just fifteen to thirty seconds to deeply reflect upon the experience of having contributed. You are compassion in action. You are life contributing to another life. Feel what it's like to be in this new state. Encode this way of engaging in life deep in your brain and nervous system.

Beyond Everyday Acts of Kindness: Contribution in the Rest of Life

It's helpful to notice everyday opportunities for contribution. But it's also important to notice the more substantial opportunities to contribute in your life. Take a step back and consider the following questions:

- Are you dedicating time, resources, or influence to a cause you believe in?
- What unique talents or abilities do you have that could enhance the lives of others?
- Are there ways that you can bring contribution into your work (mentoring, pro bono work, socially responsible initiatives, etc.)?

Your contribution will be unique because you have a distinctive set of skills, interests, and causes you believe in. You might love caring for pets or injured wild animals, or you may be interested in the environment, world or local hunger, homelessness, children's art education in your community, or HIV prevention in Africa.

Bo, a mountaineer who has reached the top of the seven

summits—the highest mountains of each of the seven continents—talks about bringing the practice of contribution into his climbs:

> *The reality of mountaineering is that we rely heavily on Sherpas and guides who live a very different life. They become members of the team, yet many of them lack the gear that they need to climb safely. So whenever I go on an expedition, I now bring extra gear. And when we are done, I give everything away. I give away my sleeping bag, my boots, my crampons, my ice axes, and just about everything else. The reaction that I get is amazing. They openly share their gratitude. And I feel grateful knowing that the Sherpas will be safer and stronger on future climbs.*

Think about the things you love to do. How could you bring contribution into these activities?

WHAT TO EXPECT

Standing before a packed crowed at the University of Portland, the Dalai Lama fielded a question from a curious student: How can a single individual change the world? The Dalai Lama didn't respond with clichés about becoming a change maker. He simply said, "Just as ripples spread out when a single pebble is dropped into water, the actions of individuals can have far-reaching effects."[16]

His words point to something profound. You can change the world through your contributions, but you may never see the changes you create. Each action—good or bad—has far-reaching effects. Complimenting a salesclerk, expressing appreciation to a family member, or donating money to a local charity—these actions create a ripple. The ripple extends even more quickly in the digital realm of email, texting, and social media. It is worth remembering that your actions can have profound effects on the lives of others in a matter of seconds. Praise and kindness travels with the same lightning-fast speed as judgment, sarcasm, and insult. Whether in real space or online, your actions instigate a sequence of changes that expands far beyond you.

Eric talks about the lasting effects of an offhand comment made by his first boss:

My first boss took me aside one morning during my first week of work and gave me a piece of great advice. "Work hard, show initiative, and be fearless. Have impact." I wasn't immediately sure what he meant by "be fearless" and asked him to clarify. "Experiment," he said. "Try to stretch yourself and seek new ways to have impact. As an entry-level employee, you really can't screw things up too badly!" I'm sure he wouldn't even remember giving me this great counsel, or possibly even remember me at all. But his advice has had a profound effect on my life. I took his interest in me to heart and did my best to follow his advice. The confidence I gained in those early years helped launch my career and put me in a position to offer the same advice to countless other young people starting their careers.

Nate had a similar experience, where a small act of contribution from his favorite college professor changed the course of his life:

His name was Ray McDermott, a professor of education at Stanford. I'll never forget walking into his class for the first time and seeing him sitting in front of us, with his puffy white hair and white beard. At the time, I was an undergrad with no clue as to what I wanted to do. I loved philosophy but wasn't sure I was good enough to pursue it as a career. Ray helped change all that, and my life, with one small act: He invited me to coffee. For forty-five minutes on a sunny Palo Alto day, Ray took an interest in me. He listened to my ideas. He invited me to collaborate with him on a project about philosophy, education, and jazz. That moment sparked a chain of events. I felt more confident in my classes and experienced a surge of motivation. Two years later, I gained admission to many of the top PhD programs in the country. Seven years later, I landed my first academic position as a professor of philosophy. When I called Ray up recently to ask if he remembered that pivotal life-changing moment, he joked, "No. I didn't even want to talk to you that day. I just like drinking coffee."

If you think back on your past, you probably have similar stories to tell—moments where a small act of contribution from a mentor, adviser, or teacher changed the course of your life. This is the way most acts of contribution work, without public recognition or even knowledge of the extent to which your actions had an impact on others.

So as you begin turning contribution into a regular habit, focus on the giving—on the small and large opportunities to improve the lives of others that occur. You may never know the full impact of these actions. But you can expect to feel a subtle shift in your own life. The more you give, the more you will inspire others around you. In turn, you will feel a deep sense of meaning emerge in your own life. And as your life takes on a deeper sense of meaning, you can expect to experience improvements in wellbeing at all levels.

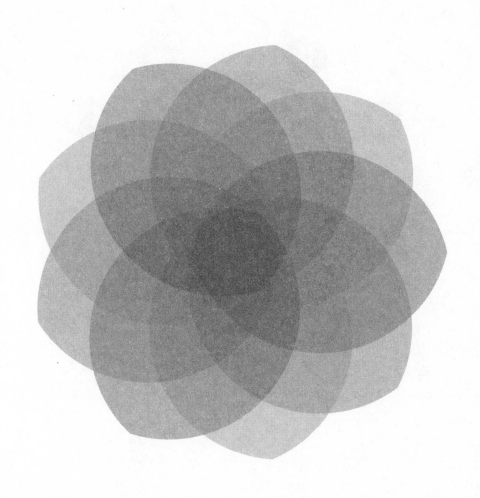

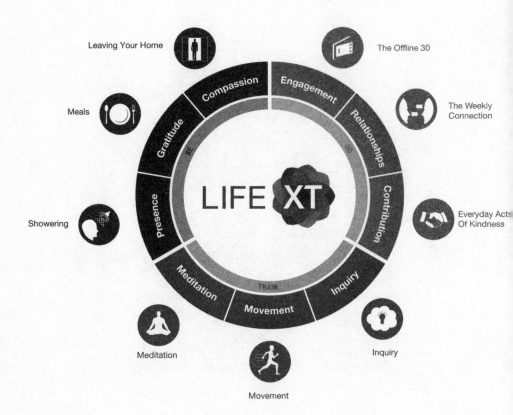

Leaving Your Home

The Offline 30

Meals

The Weekly
Connection

Showering

Everyday Acts
Of Kindness

Meditation

Movement

Inquiry

Compassion

Engagement

Gratitude

Relationships

BE

DO

Presence

LIFE XT

Contribution

Meditation

Movement

Inquiry

TRAIN

HOW TO PRACTICE LIFE CROSS TRAINING

To make things easy, we have put everything you need to practice LIFE XT in this final how-to section. What you have read thus far outlines the background, ancient wisdom, and modern science you need to understand how the practices work. This chapter provides all the practical information you need to begin building these habits, including an overview of each practice, tips, time recommendations, and suggestions for how to modify each practice if it's too much or not enough.

We encourage you to use this section along with the practice chapters as a "reference manual" for wellbeing. Participants in the LIFE XT program report that their practice improves each time they consult the how-to section for tips or reread one of the practice chapters.

A Practical Overview of LIFE XT

LIFE XT offers a road map for training nine new habits of lifelong wellbeing. We recommend beginning with a nine-week start to the program, adding one new practice each week. If you prefer to take more time with each practice, we encourage you to modify the program, taking a slower approach. If one practice is especially rewarding or challenging, feel free to extend it to several weeks or even a month. There is nothing sacred about the weekly progression. What matters is daily practice.

Each week you will focus on building one new habit. Think of it like learning a new exercise at the gym. By focusing for a week on Presence, Gratitude, and other LIFE XT habits, you establish and strengthen new neural pathways in the brain and begin strengthening the muscles of wellbeing.

To begin LIFE XT, we strongly recommend that you start with the first three Train Stage practices and that you continue these practices throughout the program. These are the foundational practices that stabilize your mind and train the skill of focused attention. They are the most fundamental to your wellbeing. As you layer on Meditation, Movement, and Inquiry over the first three weeks, do so in a way that allows you to engage in these practices every day. Once they become daily habits, you will be ready to venture on to the Be and Do Stages. Remember that the practices in these final two stages are designed for maximum efficiency. They are effective life habits you can use to shift toward a more optimal state as you move throughout your day.

You can approach building the habits in the Be and Do Stages in two different ways: the *cumulative approach* and the *cross-training approach*.

The Cumulative Approach

To add the LIFE XT habits and rituals to your life as quickly as possible, use the cumulative approach, which follows a weekly transition in which you build each habit into your daily life as you progress.

LIFE XT Cumulative Training Schedule

Week 1. Train: Meditation

- *Initial Assessment.* Complete the LIFE XT Assessment. Review your dashboard results.
- *Add Meditation.* Begin practicing breath-centered meditation (ten minutes per day).

Week 2. Train: Movement

- *Add Movement.* Exercise aerobically three times a week for at least thirty minutes and do one nonaerobic workout.

Week 3. Train: Inquiry

- *Add Inquiry.* Question one stressful thought each day immediately before or after meditation.

Week 4. Be: Presence

- *Assessment.* Complete the LIFE XT Assessment. Review your progress along all of the key dimensions of wellbeing over the first three weeks.
- *Add Presence.* Use showering as the cue to Notice-Shift-Rewire to Presence.

Week 5. Be: Gratitude

- *Add Gratitude.* Use sitting down to meals as the cue to Notice-Shift-Rewire the habit of Gratitude.

Week 6. Be: Compassion

- *Add Compassion.* Use leaving the house as the cue to Notice-Shift-Rewire the habit of Compassion.

Week 7. Do: Engagement

- *Assessment.* Complete the LIFE XT Assessment. Review your progress along all of the key dimensions of wellbeing over the first six weeks.
- *Add Engagement.* Build the Offline 30 ritual into each workday.

(continued on next page)

Week 8. Do: Relationships

- *Add Relationships.* Build the Weekly Connection ritual into each week.

Week 9. Do: Contribution

- *Add Contribution.* Build the Everyday Acts of Kindness kindness ritual into each week.
- *Final Assessment.* Complete the LIFE XT Assessment. Review your progress along all of the key dimensions of happiness and wellbeing over the first nine weeks.

The cumulative method requires considerable discipline. However, at the end of nine weeks, you will have developed a regular practice of Meditation, Movement, and Inquiry. You will be developing the three habits of Being (Presence, Gratitude, and Compassion) through your daily cues. And you will be working the three rituals of Doing (Engagement, Relationships, and Contribution) into your everyday life.

If you are ambitious and feel ready to commit, we encourage you to follow the cumulative approach. We assure you that, in time, the practices will become integrated into your daily life. Here's what a weekly training log might look like at the end of nine weeks:

Cumulative Approach (sample training schedule)

	Monday	Tuesday	Wednesday	Thursday	Friday	Saturday	Sunday
Meditation	10 min	10 min	10 min	10 min	10 min	10 min	10 min
Movement	30 min		30 min		30 min		Yoga
Inquiry	1 thought	1 thought	1 thought	1 thought	1 thought	1 thought	1 thought
Presence	X	X	X	X	X	X	X
Gratitude	X	X	X	X	X	X	X
Compassion	X	X	X	X	X	X	X
Engagement	X	X	X	X	X	X	
Relationships						X	
Contribution			X				

Note that the reason there is only one "X" in the Relationships and Contribution row is that these are weekly practices.

The Cross-Training Approach

If you elect to take a more gradual path, consider what we call the *cross-training approach*.

LIFE XT Cross-Training Schedule

Week 1. Train: Meditation

- *Initial Assessment.* Complete the LIFE XT Assessment. Review your dashboard results.
- *Add Meditation.* Begin practicing breath-centered meditation (ten minutes per day).

Week 2. Train: Movement

- *Add Movement.* Exercise aerobically three times a week for at least thirty minutes and do one nonaerobic workout.

Week 3. Train: Inquiry

- *Add Inquiry.* Question one stressful thought each day before meditation.

Week 4. Onward

- *Assessment.* Complete the LIFE XT Assessment. Review progress along all of the key dimensions of wellbeing over the first three weeks.
- *Focus on one or more Be or Do Stage practices each month.*
- *Continue completing the LIFE XT Assessment every three to four weeks.*

We still encourage you to begin with a regular practice of Meditation, Movement, and Inquiry. As with the cumulative approach, you can add one of these practices each week or proceed more slowly, adding one every couple of weeks or even every month. Once you have established a strong foundation, select one or two of the Be and Do Stage habits to focus on each month. You can add these in order, rely on your own intuition, or use the online LIFE XT Assessment tool to guide you toward those habits that will offer maximum benefit based on your individual needs.

At the end of each month, switch. Choose a different practice to develop for the month ahead. Rest assured that this approach, though more deliberate, will yield powerful results. After a month of working with each practice, you will have formed the habit, and this will allow you to maintain the practice with minimal conscious effort.

Over time, this cross-training approach will lead you to the same place as the cumulative approach: You will integrate each of these habits into your everyday life. The next page shows what a weekly training log might look like if you were using the cross-training approach to focus for a month on the habit of Gratitude.

The Cross-Training Approach (sample schedule)

	Monday	Tuesday	Wednesday	Thursday	Friday	Saturday	Sunday
Meditation	10 min	10 min	10 min	10 min	10 min	10 min	10 min
Movement	30 min		30 min		30 min		Yoga
Inquiry	1 thought	1 thought	1 thought	1 thought	1 thought	1 thought	1 thought
Gratitude	X	X	X	X	X	X	X

Completing the LIFE XT Assessment

We have developed a Wellbeing Assessment tool that you can use to track your progress throughout the program. This assessment was designed in collaboration with some of the world's leading experts on measuring wellbeing—researchers like Drs. John and Stephanie Cacioppo at the University of Chicago.

Take the ten-minute assessment at the start of each of the three stages (at the beginning of weeks 1, 4, and 7), or if you are moving more slowly, take it every four weeks. This tool gives you a baseline measurement of your wellbeing set point and then shows how your happiness levels change as you progress throughout the program.

Habit 1: Meditation

Before You Start

Complete the LIFE XT Wellbeing Assessment (it should take only about ten minutes) and then review your initial results. This will give you a baseline measure of your happiness set point and overall wellbeing, quantified across twenty different metrics.

How to Do It

Start by identifying a convenient time and place to meditate. As you sit down to meditate, set a brief intention and then begin the practice of mindfully following the breath. You can either set a timer or use one of the guided meditations available at www. LIFE-XT.com. If you are new to meditation, we recommend that you gradually increase your time to ten minutes each day using this schedule:

- *Days 1 and 2:*   3 Minutes
- *Days 3 and 4:*   5 Minutes
- *Days 5 and 6:*   7 Minutes
- *Day 7:*   10 Minutes

When you are finished meditating, see if you can take this experience with you, into the rest of your day.

Quick Tips

- Remember that meditation isn't about stopping your thoughts.
- If you feel sleepy, don't judge yourself as doing it incorrectly. Pay attention to your posture. Sit upright and keep your spine erect. You can also try meditating first thing in the morning. The feeling of sleepiness usually goes away after the first few weeks.
- Find a partner to do it with you; that way, you can hold each other accountable.

- If it's just not working for you, consider finding a meditation instructor who can help guide you.
- After about a year of meditating (or sooner if you feel inspired to), consider going on a meditation retreat.

Guidelines

- *If it's too much.* Stay with three to five minutes until you feel ready to add more time.
- *If it's not enough.* Feel free to add more time to your daily meditations. We advise that you add on slowly: no more than five minutes per day.
- *If you already meditate.* Keep up the good work. Focus on maintaining consistency, and if you feel like a challenge, try lengthening your daily sessions.
- *If you are having trouble getting motivated.* Meditate for a short amount of time (three to five minutes) until you are able to build the daily habit.
- *If you get tense while meditating.* That's fine. Just notice it and try to avoid judging yourself as doing it "wrong." The key is to notice what is going on. Noticing that you are tense is, in fact, doing it right. Feeling tension is a sign that you are working too hard to direct your focus to your breath. Ideally, you should feel yourself dropping into the awareness of the breath, not forcing it. If you feel tense or anxious, focus on relaxing your body and mind with each exhalation.
- *If you get lost in mind wandering.* This is normal and happens to everyone. If, however, your mind is so busy that you can't focus, try labeling each inhale and exhale. Each time

you breathe in, make a mental note of inhale. Each time you breathe out, make a mental note of exhale. Once your attention stabilizes, you can drop the labeling and just focus on the sensation of breathing.

- *The advanced practice.* Try the advanced open awareness practice described in the chapter on meditation. You can also experiment with taking your practice off the meditation cushion and into the world. Try meditating while flying on an airplane or riding on a train. Try it in the waiting room at your doctor's office. Try it in nature or while waiting in line at the store. This integration of meditation and everyday life will help you remember that the goal isn't to become an amazing meditator. The goal is to bring this more open, relaxed awareness into the other twenty-three hours of the day.

Habit 2: Movement

How to Do It

To turn movement into a habit, start by finding a form of movement that you enjoy. Then set a realistic goal. The LIFE XT recommendation is to do some form of aerobic exercise for at least thirty minutes three times per week and do one nonaerobic workout once per week. But feel free to set your personal goal above or below this recommended amount.

Record your initial goal right now: "I will move aerobically for
_____ minutes _____ times per week and do _____ nonaerobic
workout(s)." Now, if you want to go one step further, pick up your
phone or Day-Timer and add your workouts for the next week to
your calendar.

Quick Tips

- Find a workout partner or communicate your goal to others.
  This will make it more fun and help you with accountability.
- Use a Fitbit or Jawbone device or the tracking tools available
  on the LIFE XT website.
- Start slow to minimize the risk of injury. This will also help
  you stay with it.
- *Make it social.* Invite your friends or family members to
  work out with you. Conduct meetings while walking. Come
  up with imaginative ways to turn movement into a social
  event.
- *Strive for consistency.* Exercise at the same time each day. This
  is a key to habit building. It will help you turn movement into
  a routine.
- *Develop the habit of moving throughout the day.* Take breaks
  every hour in which you get up and stretch or take a short walk.
- *Celebrate your success.*

Guidelines

- *If it's too much.* Lower your goal to fifteen or even ten minutes
  three times per week.

- *If it's not enough.* You may already have a workout program that far exceeds the recommended goal. If that's the case, stick with it and work on integrating the advanced LIFE XT prescription: Do something different one day per week. If you run every day, do yoga or Pilates. If you do yoga daily, go on a long hike once a week.
- *If you can't get motivated.* Make a deal with yourself: *All I have to do is put my exercise gear on and work out for five minutes. Then I can stop if I want.* Ninety-eight percent of the time, once you've started, you will keep going beyond the five minutes.
- *Not sure whether you should favor moderate or more intense forms of exercise?* Try both and see what happens when you alternate between the two. If that's too much, then go for more moderate forms of aerobic movement. If you love the intensity, then add more vigorous forms of movement.
- *When should you stop?* Exercise places stress on the body, which in the beginning, you will feel in the form of dull, sometimes achy sensations in the muscles throughout the body. This is normal. If, on the other hand, you start to feel sharper sensations—tweaks, joint pain, or nerve pain—surfacing during or after your workouts, it's a sign that you need to decrease the intensity of the exercise or try something different.

How to Incorporate Movement into Your Work

As you know from the Movement chapter, exercise is only one part of the movement equation. To experience the full benefits of the practice, we recommend that you begin building movement into the rest of your everyday life. Of course, your job may require you to stay in one place most of the time, use a computer, or attend meetings. But even in these situations, there are a few easy ways to add movement to your day and counter the harmful effects of sedentary behavior:

- *Take frequent breaks.* If your job requires sitting, then schedule regular movement breaks throughout the day. Get up, walk up a flight of stairs, do a lap around your building, or stretch. The goal is to break your body out of the sedentary state.

- *Stand.* In response to the growing body of research on the effects of our modern lifestyle, we have seen the rise of new inventions like the convertible desk, the standing desk, and the treadmill desk. These new takes on the traditional workspace allow you to shift out of the sedentary life by standing (or walking)—an activity that burns around sixty more calories per hour than sitting. If you don't have a standing workspace, try standing whenever you talk on the phone or whenever you check texts or emails on your phone. It's also worth noting that, while standing has important benefits, it is possible to stand too much. Jack Callaghan, a researcher in kinesiology, found that excessive standing led to lower back pain in 50 percent of those who participated in a study on the effects of standing at the workplace.[1] Other researchers have shown that excessive standing places an excessive load on the circulatory system, which increases the risk of varicose veins.[2] Given the problems associated with excessive standing, Callaghan recommends a 1:1 ratio of alternating between twenty and thirty minutes of sitting and standing throughout the day.

- *Do the television workout.* For many of us, our most sedentary hours are those spent watching TV. After a long day, the temptation is to sit back on the couch or in a chair and relax. Remember, this is a habit. To break the habit, make the following deal with yourself: *Whenever I watch TV, I need to be moving.* Or if that is too ambitious, you might commit to moving during commercials. Watching television is the perfect time for core work: sit-ups, crunches, and other core-strengthening exercises. It is also the perfect time for stretching, increasing the flexibility of your hamstrings, neck, and shoulders.

Habit 3: Inquiry

How to Do It

Inquiry requires that we set aside focused time and go inward to reflect. Start by identifying a stressful thought to question. If you are having trouble or just want a deeper experience of Inquiry, use the Judge Your Neighbor Worksheet (available for free at www.TheWork.com). Questions one through five will help you generate a list of stressful thoughts to question. Once you have identified the thought, it's time to begin the process of Inquiry. When asking yourself the four questions and turnaround of The Work, you can write out your responses on index cards or, if you would like a more guided experience, print out the One-Belief-at-a-Time Worksheet (also available for free at www.TheWork.com).

The next step is to meditate on and write out your answers to the four questions:

1. Is it true?
2. Can you absolutely know that it's true?
3. How do you react—what happens—when you believe that thought?
4. Who would you be without the thought?

The final step is to turn the thought around (consider its opposite) and write down at least three specific, genuine examples of how each turnaround is true for you in this situation.

Your goal will be to inquire on at least one thought each day.

Quick Tips

- *Do it with a friend.* Although it works well to write out your responses, many people find that practicing Inquiry with a partner enhances the experience. Have one person ask the questions while the other answers, and then switch.
- *Track your Inquiry practice.*
- *Be consistent.* Try to practice Inquiry at the same time each day. We have found that it works well to combine Inquiry and Meditation. Before you meditate, question your most stressful thought.
- If you are struggling with the practice or want to go deeper, go to Byron Katie's website (www.TheWork.com) to view videos of her doing Inquiry with people on a wide range of challenges.

Guidelines

- *If it's too much.* Try practicing Inquiry at different times. Once you find a time that works well, build a habit by doing it every day at that time.
- *If it's not enough.* You can always question more than one thought each day. We have also found that adding one deep dive into inquiry each week powerfully accelerates your progress. Each week, set aside thirty minutes or an hour to practice inquiry. It's even better if you can do it a beautiful setting—on a hilltop, at the beach, in your yard or a park, or by the fireplace. During this time, question each stressful thought that arises. As you work through a number of interconnected stressful thoughts, this practice will cultivate an even deeper sense of freedom.

More Guidance on How to Approach Each Question

The four questions and the turnaround offer a helpful road map for questioning your thoughts. But it can also be helpful to consider a few practical pointers for each part of the process.

- *Preparing for Inquiry.* Before you begin asking the questions, remind yourself to slow down and do inquiry without a motive. Then identify a specific situation when you experienced stress as a result of the thought. Bring the situation to mind and answer each of the questions from that moment in time.

- *Question 1. Is it true?* This is an essential question because it helps you notice the thought as a thought, creating a subtle sense of separation between you and the thought. In time, this question becomes the shorthand for the entire sequence. When you experience a stressful thought, you simply pop this question, and the stress unwinds.

- *Question 2. Can you absolutely know that it's true?* Your initial answer might feel like yes, but even when a thought feels completely true, this question makes you hold out the possibility that a stressful thought is just that—a stressful *thought*, not reality.

- *Question 3. How do you react—what happens—when you believe that thought?* Once you have isolated the thought, this question requires you to experience the felt emotions associated with it. By watching the waves of negative emotion and thought loops that spring from simply bringing the thought into consciousness, you see how the thought grips you and can begin the process of developing some space around it. If you are questioning a judgment about another person, be sure to consider both how you react toward yourself and how you react toward them in the situation.

- *Question 4. Who would you be without the thought?* Return to the stressful situation and notice how an immediate sense of peace breaks out when you reflect on this question. You experience a radical contrast between the stress of believing the thought and the peace of letting it go. You feel a sense of space between you and the thought-created disturbances floating across your mind. Notice how you feel, how you react, and how you treat others when you can no longer believe the thought.

- *Turnaround.* The turnaround is the power move that sets you free. When you generate each of the three turnarounds (to the self, to the other, and to the opposite), you find that proof is always available. You see that the opposite of virtually anything you could think could also be true. You're led to the place that the ancients called *not-knowing, the beginner's mind,* or *knowing that you don't know.* You become freed from the thought-generated limits of the mind.

What to Do When You Finish Questioning Each Belief

When you are done with the questions and the turnaround, be sure to savor the experience of wellbeing that arises. You can also identify what Byron Katie calls a "Living Turnaround." This is a turnaround that you will take off the worksheet and into your life. The practice is straightforward. Take the turnaround that generated the most profound shift in your thinking and live it for the day. If the thought is *My spouse doesn't pay enough attention to me,* the living turnaround might be *I don't pay enough attention to my spouse.* The practice would then be to live that turnaround for the day—to spend the rest of the day following the advice of the turnaround by consciously paying more attention to your spouse. This will help you keep the practice of Inquiry alive throughout each day.

Habit 4: Presence

Before You Start

Now that you are a third of the way through the program, it is a good time to take the LIFE XT Wellbeing Assessment again. You will now be able to see specific areas of improvement on your wellbeing dashboard.

How to Do It

Use showering as your cue to Notice-Shift-Rewire to the present moment. Notice—see if you can become aware—each time you step into the shower. Shift your attention to the sights, sounds, and sensations of the present moment. Feel the warmth of the water; hear the sounds it makes when it hits the floor and other surfaces. Notice the feeling of the shampoo suds between your fingers as you wash your hair.

Quick Tips

- Track your daily Presence practice.
- Practice presence every day and, if you forget to do it in the shower, Notice-Shift-Rewire to presence during some other

everyday life moment, such as walking up the stairs or starting your car.

- Pretend each shower is your last. Imagine if today was your
  last day alive. How would the shower feel?

Guidelines

- *How to remember to do it.* The most difficult thing about building this habit is remembering. To help you remember, we
  have developed a low-tech but extremely effective method.
  Put a sticker at eye level on your shower door. If you don't
  want to use a sticker (or don't have a shower door), you could
  use a piece of masking tape with *Presence* or *NSR* written on
  it. After a month or so, once the habit is ingrained, you may
  find that you no longer need it.

- *Pretend each shower is your first.* This is a new way of showering. See if you can enter each day with total freshness of
  mind—what the Zen tradition calls *beginner's mind.* Imagine
  you are studying the sensations that arise as you first stand
  under the stream of water. Notice the smells, the sounds, and
  the sensations that arise. Feel like you are witnessing the experience of showering for the first time.

- *How you know it's working.* After a couple of weeks or a
  month, you will likely start to notice that you no longer need
  to consciously remember to experience presence. It just starts
  to happen as you enter the shower. This is the magic moment
  of habit formation. It means that your brain has wired a new
  set of connections around this everyday life activity.

- *If showering isn't a good cue for you.* Choose some other daily
  life event if showering doesn't work for you. Here are a few

possibilities: brushing your teeth, getting out of your car, making or buying your morning beverage. The key is to use the same cue every day. The goal, after all, is habit formation, and to do this effectively, it is essential to use a consistent cue.

- *If you want more.* If you have mastered the habit of Notice-Shift-Rewire in the shower, try adding the advanced LIFE XT cue: stairs. Every time you walk up or down a flight of stairs, see if you can Notice-Shift-Rewire to presence. This is a perfect time to feel the sensations in your feet or to bring your attention to the sights and sounds that occur as you step. This additional cue will take you even deeper into the experience of presence.

Habit 5: Gratitude

How to Do It

Use meals as your cue to Notice-Shift-Rewire to gratitude. Notice each time you sit down to eat. Shift by redirecting your attention to gratitude. If you are alone, take a moment to think about a few things that you are grateful for in that moment. If you are with friends, family, or coworkers, you might ask them what they are grateful for. Then give each person the opportunity to express one thing that he or she is grateful for in that moment. Rewire by taking a few seconds to savor your feelings of gratitude.

Quick Tips

- Track your daily Gratitude practice.
- Get your friends and family involved. Have each person say what he or she is grateful for at the start of a meal. This will reinforce the experience and help everyone remember to do it.
- Email your gratitude. Send a quick note to a friend, a family member, or a coworker expressing appreciation. Chances are you will make their day.
- Do it every day, and if you forget to Notice-Shift-Rewire to gratitude at the beginning of a meal, do it during some other everyday moment during the day.

Guidelines

- *How to remember to do it.* Like all of the Be Stage habits, the most difficult part of the Gratitude practice is remembering. We recommend two strategies. First, as mentioned above, get your family and friends involved. When you sit down to eat, each of you will help one another remember. Second, you can use the sticker technique. Put a small sticker with *NSR* or *Gratitude* written on it in the upper corner of your place mat. This will give you a visual reminder each time you eat at home.
- *Don't forget to rewire.* It's natural to experience gratitude in one instant and then move on to eating or whatever else you are doing in the next. Remember to introduce a subtle space after gratitude. For just fifteen seconds, savor the experience—feel yourself taking in the good.

- *How you know it's working.* In a few weeks or a month, when you sit down to eat, you will express and savor your gratitudes for the day automatically. You will also start to notice the experience of gratitude becoming more frequent in the rest of your life.

- *If meals aren't a good cue for you.* We strongly recommend meals because they often involve social situations in which you can share your gratitude with others. But if this cue doesn't work for you, feel free to pick some other, regularly repeated daily event: waking up, going to bed, or starting your computer at the beginning of the day. The key is to keep your cue consistent.

- *If you want more.* If you have mastered the practice of expressing gratitude at each meal, then feel free to begin building the advanced cue into your daily life: phone calls. Whenever you receive a phone call, rather than picking it up immediately, listen to at least two rings while thinking of one thing you are grateful for, and then answer the call as you savor the experience. You will find this practice more difficult than it sounds. When you master it, it will enable you to enter each phone conversation with a feeling of deep appreciation. It will also remind you of the power of Notice-Shift-Rewire again and again as you move throughout each day.

Habit 6: Compassion

How to Do It

To build this daily habit, use leaving your home each day as your cue to Notice-Shift-Rewire to compassion. Notice each time you leave your house or apartment, whether you are headed to work or just headed to the store to pick up groceries. Shift by redirecting your attention to compassion. As you walk out the door, think of all the people you will come in contact with that day and take a moment to feel compassion toward them. You can do this by flooding your body with a feeling of warmth for these people or thinking to yourself, *May everyone I come in contact with today be happy.* Rewire by taking a few seconds to savor this flood of loving-kindness.

Quick Tips

- Track your daily Compassion practice.
- Build in some social support by getting friends or family members involved in the practice.
- If you forget to Notice-Shift-Rewire to compassion on your way out of the house, pick some other life moment to experience compassion: checking out at the store, sitting in traffic, or talking to a stranger on the phone.

Guidelines

- *How to remember to do it.* The most difficult thing about this practice is simply remembering to do it as you leave your home each day. When you first start, your mind has no association between walking out the door and compassion. You will need to build that. As with Presence and Gratitude, the sticker technique works well for many people. Put a small sticker with NSR or Compassion written on it at eye level on the frame of the door you use to leave the house. This will give you a visual reminder each time you leave home.

- *Don't forget to rewire.* It is important to savor the experience of compassion for just a few seconds. If you drive a car, the moment before you start the ignition is a perfect time for this. Feel compassion as you leave the house and then savor it as you get settled in the driver's seat. If you don't drive, choose some other cue for savoring: walking along the sidewalk, waiting at the bus stop, or taking the stairs to the subway station.

- *If leaving the house isn't a good cue for you.* We have found leaving the house to be a powerful cue for developing the habit of compassion. But if you work from home or travel frequently and want to choose a different cue, just be sure that you pick something that you do every day, such as brushing your teeth at night. Conjure up the images of all the people you encountered during the day and extend the feeling of compassion toward them as they prepare to sleep. And of course stick with this cue. That's the key to forming the habit.

- *If you want more.* If you have mastered the practice of experiencing compassion when you leave your home and you want more, feel free to begin building the advanced cue into your daily life: good-byes. Most of us say good-bye to family members, friends, and coworkers throughout the day. And yet rarely, if ever, do we pay close attention to these moments. The advanced practice is to feel deep compassion every time you say good-bye to someone. When you kiss your partner on the way out the door, when you hug your child on his way to school, or when you say good-bye to your coworker at the end of the day, see if you can feel a sense of loving-kindness toward the person. Soon your entire life will serve as a reminder to feel compassion.

- *How to fit in compassion meditation.* Like the breath-centered meditation you learned in the chapter on meditation, compassion meditation requires that you set aside time for it. Instead of trying to do both breath-centered meditation and compassion meditation, we recommend focusing solely on compassion meditation for a couple of weeks or even a month. Do this at the same time of day for the same amount of time as your previous practice. Once you feel comfortable with compassion meditation, feel free to alternate between your breath-centered focused attention practice and compassion meditation.

Habit 7: Engagement

Before You Start

Now that you are two-thirds of the way through the program, it is a good time to take the LIFE XT Wellbeing Assessment again. You will now be able to see specific areas of improvement on your wellbeing dashboard.

How to Do It

The LIFE XT Engagement practice is a ritual that you can build into each day. We call this ritual the Offline 30. Each day reserve thirty minutes (or more) for engaged and undistracted work. Shut down or mute your phone, close your browser and email, and turn off the TV. Do whatever you need to do to eliminate the countless digital distractions that call for your attention. This straightforward and effective practice will enhance wellbeing on all levels, helping you become less distracted and more focused, productive, and inspired.

Quick Tips

- Track your daily Engagement practice.
- Turn off *everything*. If you really want to free yourself from distractions during this practice, close down all the programs on your computer that might tempt you—email, web browser, social media, etc.
- To remind yourself to sprint and recover by taking occasional breaks throughout the day, consider using a timer or a free Pomodoro Timer app (a popular break-reminder system) to remind you when it's time to take a break.

Guidelines

- *How to remember to do it.* Schedule the Offline 30. Put it in your calendar for every workday. If something comes up, you can always move it. But for many people, it is more likely to get done if it's on their calendar.
- *How to bring it into your workplace.* If you work with a larger team in a company or organization, see if you can convince your coworkers to play along. Schedule a time each day that is free from meetings, calls, email, and other distractions. You will likely find a significant shift in productivity and creative insight throughout the organization.
- *If you want more.* Thirty minutes is a great place to start. But when it comes to engagement, more is better. As you build this habit, try creating an Offline 60 or even an Offline 120. If, however, you extend this time of full engagement beyond 90 to 120 minutes, remember the principle of sprint and recover.

Working at peak intensity for eight hours straight isn't possible. So as you add time, be sure to also add periods of recovery.

How to Sprint and Recover in Everyday Life

For those who work from home or own their own business, adopting this habit is relatively straightforward: Just use your calendar, a timer, or an app to help you remember to add more breaks to your day. If you are like most people, however, and you work at a job, you might be thinking, *The idea of sprint and recover sounds great, but how am I supposed to do this at work? I can't work for just 90 minutes and then start doing stretches!*

The underlying challenge here is that most workplaces are set up on the marathon model of work—the idea that you achieve maximum productivity by sitting in one place all day without taking breaks. So in building this habit, you will have to be a bit more skillful in how you alternate between periods of maximum focus and periods of recovery. Here are a couple of tips:

- *Sequence your work.* Some work (writing, creative thinking, delivering presentations, etc.) requires total engagement and deep focus. Some work (filing, cleaning up your desk, organizing, and even emailing) requires minimal focus. One of the best things you can do to maximize engagement is start with your most demanding, high-intensity tasks. You can then use lower intensity tasks as periods of recovery.

- *Take creative breaks.* If you work at a desk, make a habit of getting up at least once every hour (remember all the benefits from the chapter on movement). Use these breaks as conscious moments of recovery. As you walk around the office, be present and let yourself relax into the break. You can also use many of the practices of LIFE XT to give yourself a break: Experience gratitude, feel compassion, or do a mini-meditation.

Habit 8: Relationships

How to Do It

The LIFE XT Relationships practice involves building a simple yet extremely powerful ritual into your everyday life—the Weekly Connection. Most of us already spend significant amounts of time in the physical presence of people we love. But simply being *with* someone isn't the same as being *connected to* the people we love. The Weekly Connection is your invitation to break out of the ordinary patterns of busyness and distraction. The practice is straightforward: Schedule one time each week to experience quality time with someone you love.

Quick Tips

- Track your weekly Relationships practice.
- Use your calendar. Each month, schedule times in your calendar to take your spouse out to dinner, to walk with a friend, or to take your child to a baseball game.

- Set a monthly or even weekly reminder to help you remember to schedule time with your loved ones.

Guidelines

- *Have fun.* Of all the practices of LIFE XT, the Weekly Connection is the easiest and most fun, so be sure not to turn it into a burden. These weekly connections can become a great part of your week—an opportunity to unwind and enjoy the company of someone you love.
- *If you want more.* Once a week is a perfect place to start. If you want more, schedule as many times for connection as you choose.

Ways to Notice-Shift-Rewire in Your Relationships Throughout the Day

The Weekly Connection is the starting point. The more advanced practice is to savor your relationships throughout the course of each day. Here are a few tips for building this skill deeper into your everyday life:

- *Listen.* Being present with another person requires mastering the skill of listening. As you talk with your friends and family, be present with them. Soak in their experience. Make it about them, not about you.
- *Appreciate.* Another way to shift toward presence in relationships is through appreciation. When a friend or a romantic partner tells you about a hard day, appreciate them

for who they are in this moment—for their openness, their strength, or their vulnerability. When your son walks off the field, appreciate him for his tenacity, grit, or attitude. Appreciations draw everyone around you into presence. Offering appreciation helps you become present to the gifts of others.

- *Stay curious and inquire.* If presence is important in moments of ease, it's essential in moments of conflict. Few relationships are immune from conflict. It's something that inevitably happens when you love someone deeply. In these moments, we tend to overestimate our inputs to the relationship and underestimate those of the other person. It's easy to see why this happens. You know exactly how many times you've cleaned up after your partner or paid a bill for them. You have much less knowledge of all the things the other person has done for you. By shifting to curiosity, you shift away from this habitual tendency to favor your own point of view. Curiosity helps you stay present. It will help you work through conflicts by focusing on love and empathy, rather than resentment (the past) or fear (the future). If you like, use these conflict-related thoughts as thoughts you use in your daily Inquiry practice.

Habit 9: Contribution

How to Do It

This final LIFE XT practice will help you turn contribution into a regular part of your life. We call it Everyday Acts of Kindness. The goal is to make these acts of generosity and service a weekly or even daily ritual. You don't need to donate millions or save someone's life for your act to matter. A simple and small kind act that improves the life of a fellow being is all that is required. The field of possibilities is limitless. You could pick up a piece of trash off the sidewalk. You could pay the toll for the driver behind you. You could allow a rushed traveler to move ahead of you in an airport security line.

Quick Tips

- Track your weekly Contribution practice.
- Enlist social support. See if you can find one other person to take on the weekly Everyday Acts of Kindness challenge with you.
- Mix it up. Do something different each day or week. Contribute at home one week, at the office the next, at the grocery store the next, and so on.

Guidelines

- *Start small.* At the beginning, focus on small, easy-to-complete spontaneous acts of kindness. These can be everyday acts that take minimal time to complete but improve the lives of others: giving a few dollars to someone in need, offering your place in line to someone else, or cooking dinner for your spouse.

- *If you can't remember.* Designate one day each week as "contribution day." Put it in your calendar or schedule a repeating weekly notification on your phone. Do whatever you need to do to start the day with the intention of giving to another person.

- *Bring it into your workplace.* In our work with companies, we have found that the Contribution practice becomes even more meaningful and fun when others are involved. At work, consider creating a contribution challenge. Divide the office into teams and have a friendly competition to see which team can complete the most random acts of kindness.

- *Don't forget to savor.* As in all LIFE XT practices, be sure to take a brief moment to rewire this experience of contribution. For just fifteen seconds, feel the shift in your mental, emotional, and physical experience.

- *If you want more.* Do one everyday act of kindness every day or even multiple times a day. You can also direct your attention to the questions listed in the "Beyond Everyday Acts of Kindness" section of the Contribution chapter. They will help you integrate this practice of contribution at a deeper level. You will begin to reflect on the importance of giving to a cause you believe in and more effectively using your career as an opportunity to contribute to the lives of others.

LIFE XT for Life

At the End of All Nine Habits

Take the LIFE XT Wellbeing Assessment again and continue to do so every three months. You will be able to see specific areas of improvement on your wellbeing dashboard. Draw your attention to the areas that have changed the most and congratulate yourself on your progress.

What Do I Do Now?

You have now developed a new set of lifelong habits for wellbeing. With time, you will find that you look forward to your three daily Train practices and will naturally prioritize these over other activities. You will also find that it becomes easier and easier to seamlessly integrate the six Be and Do practices into your life.

Integrating Life Cross Training into Your Life

In the process of developing LIFE XT, we spent years integrating these practices into our lives. We have also shared these practices with thousands of people at some of the country's leading businesses, including top law firms, digital media agencies, financial institutions, consulting firms, and venture capital firms. All have shared an interest in elevating themselves to peak performance and shared a desire to become more resilient and experience better emotional health.

Our lives, like those of every other LIFE XT practitioner, aren't perfect. But over time, through the LIFE XT Assessment, we have measured profound and wonderful shifts in people's wellbeing and experience of life. We have found that in a matter of months these practices lead to measurable results:

- 33 percent rise in satisfaction with life
- 23 percent increase in resiliency to stress
- 23 percent rise in satisfaction with relationships
- 16 percent increase in focus[1]

We encourage you to test this for yourself and measure your own progress along the way.

The Skill of Wellbeing

You have now reached a crossroads in your LIFE XT journey and the start of a new way of being. As the poet T. S. Eliot once wrote, "And to make an end is to make a beginning. / The end is where we start from."[2] Nowhere is this truer than in the inner journey of LIFE XT. As you have learned, training the skill of lifelong wellbeing is not just about reading a book, nor is it about experiencing these practices for nine weeks and then returning to old habits. The program is focused on a much larger goal: cultivating lifelong habits that give you a new way of living and taking action in the world.

As you continue your daily practice over the coming months and years, keep in mind these three core insights that run throughout all of LIFE XT:

- *Wellbeing is a skill that can be trained.* Our habits of thought and action may be strong, but they aren't fixed. Recall Donald Hebb's inspiring adage of modern neuroscience: "Neurons that fire together, wire together." We each have the power to alter even the most deeply entrenched habits that keep us feeling less than fulfilled, continuously stressed, frustrated, and living with a background sense of unease. Reshaping these long-standing habits and thought patterns requires a disciplined commitment to cross-training the mind.
- *Choosing where we direct our attention defines our experience.* Recall these words of William James: "My experience is what I agree to attend to."[3] By learning to direct our attention to more positive and productive ends, we shape our inner experience. Whether we follow our ordinary and unconscious habits of mind or shift to presence, gratitude, or compassion

defines our life experience. How we engage in our work, invest in our relationships, and contribute to the world creates our reality. LIFE XT provides the tools to develop this life-changing muscle of attention.

- *Every moment in everyday life offers an opportunity to shift.* LIFE XT's mind training isn't something you do for twenty minutes at the beginning of the day and then forget about. It is a moment-to-moment practice: something you do in the shower, at dinner, or on your way out the door. Each new moment presents an opportunity to strengthen the habit of Notice-Shift-Rewire—to build the Be and Do Stage practices deep into your everyday experience life. You don't need to go on a monthlong retreat or move to the woods to integrate these practices into your life and experience their benefits. The ordinary activities of everyday life provide an ample training ground.

Three Tips

As you develop your LIFE XT practice over the coming months and years, use these three tips to help you get the most out of your efforts:

- *Track and assess your progress.* The LIFE XT program is designed to keep track of your progress and to help you measure the extent to which these practices have become habits. As you continue, we recommend that you continue using the Wellbeing Assessment each month to measure your progress and identify your strengths and weaknesses. The tracking tools will help you stay motivated and help hold you accountable to your practice goals. The assessment tool will enable you to see the specific benefits arising from your practice and will give you detailed insight into how to improve your practice.

- *Find a LIFE XT community.* Creating a LIFE XT community is perhaps the best way to ensure that you see powerful results. The first and most important step is to find a training partner, another person who will take the LIFE XT journey along with you. This partnership will become an invaluable source of inspiration and support along the way. It will give you someone to share your victories with and someone to encourage you during the tough times.

- *Read and reread. Start Here* is meant to be a life manual— a kind of Lonely Planet guide for the soul. If you just finished reading the book, the insights and practice tips in the book will be fresh and relatively easy to recall. As the weeks, months, or even years go by, however, you will begin to forget these essential facts. This has certainly been our experience— and we did the research and wrote the book. So it's worth revisiting the practice chapters to refresh your understanding of each of these practices. As your mastery of these skills evolves and your experience of the practices deepens, each time you reread a chapter, you will likely understand it in a different way, and it will continue to inspire, inform, and motivate you to continue training the core skills of wellbeing.

Opening Beyond the Secret

We began *Start Here* with the Open Secret—the idea that beneath the polished facade others may project, everyone experiences a level of pain, fear, and dissatisfaction. It's a truth worth repeating because it's so easy to forget. Each time we log on to Facebook, attend a dinner party, or turn on the TV, we see glistening smiles, fabulous vacations, and inspiring achievements. We can begin to think that everyone has it together—except for us.

By now it should be clear that this just isn't the case. Everyone experiences the very same set point forces of the mind. We have all felt the sting of judgment, the grip of attachment, and the white-knuckled dread of resistance. In the privacy of our own minds, we are all experts on this biological predisposition toward anxiety, vigilance, and negative thinking.

Returning to this theme in the final pages of the book is meant to remind you of the well-worn cliché that life is a journey. As you well know by now, you will have good days and bad days, great years and harder years. The ultimate value of a program like LIFE XT is that it gives you a road map and the most efficient methodology for navigating this journey. It's a set of tools that will help you optimize your sense of wellbeing during the good times and help you get back on your feet during times of intense stress or challenging life changes.

It's not a matter of whether we will encounter these moments but a matter of when. And in these times, we have two responses available to us. The first is to allow our old habits of mind to run the show—to go on autopilot and let ourselves get hooked by drama, fear, irritation, and sadness. The second is to rely on a daily practice and the inner technology of Notice-Shift-Rewire to shift toward a more present, open, and accepting state. Pema Chödrön offers a perfect description of this choice: "Ordinarily," she writes, "we are swept away by habitual momentum. We don't interrupt our patterns even slightly. With practice, however . . . we learn to be cool when the ground beneath us suddenly disappears."[4]

This is what it all boils down to. In each moment, we have a choice. The challenge is that we so easily forget. This is why the framework of LIFE XT is so important to keep in your life during good times and bad. Your daily practice of meditation, movement, and inquiry will help you sustain a high level of mental, physical, and emotional fitness. And your efforts to integrate the Be and Do habits into your daily life will positively shape your experience.

When it comes to living a full and meaningful life, exercising our ability to choose is perhaps the ultimate skill. Viktor Frankl, the Austrian-born psychiatrist and Holocaust survivor, put it this way: "Everything can be taken from a man but one thing: the last of the human freedoms—to choose one's attitude in any given set of circumstances, to choose one's own way."[5]

As you begin to weave the practices of LIFE XT into your everyday life, you train this "last of the human freedoms." By choosing to shift in any given moment, you become more present, grateful, and compassionate. You become more engaged in your work, your relationships, and your service to others. You experience the sense of joy and aliveness that springs from mastering the lifelong habit of wellbeing.

Enjoy the adventure.

Acknowledgments

Our Gratitudes

Gratitude is a core LIFE XT practice. And it is how we wish to end *Start Here*. Over the many years it took us to research and write this book, we have benefited from the ideas, insights, and support of many people. In fact, we watched in awe as an entire LIFE XT community developed alongside this project.

Several key advisers helped us develop and validate the LIFE XT program. We are grateful to Drs. John and Stephanie Cacioppo for their help validating the science of LIFE XT and helping us construct the Wellbeing Assessment Tool and our overall human analytics strategy. We are grateful to Dr. Richard Davidson for his support of the project and for his constructive advice on the manuscript and program.

Our associates at LIFE XT also played an essential role. Thanks to Priti Patel, Erika Pacheco, Amanda Schleede, Jane Shepard, and Adam Smith. Along the way, many friends of LIFE XT offered powerful insights and advice. We're particularly grateful to Meaghan Benjamin, Carter Cast, Andrea Cohen, Jack and Judy Craven, Gigi Day, Bruce Doblin, Jordan Dolin, Ben Feder, Jim Gimian, Jason Girzadas, Kelsey Kates, Jacob Klein, Alexander Langshur, Avi Lewittes, Greg Makoul, Kelly O'Brien, Anne Saunders, Jeanne Talbot, Scott Ullem, and Grant Zemont.

The book and program would also not have been possible without the help of a dedicated team of business advisers and partners. In particular, we are grateful to Laura Anderson, Michael Cole, Manish Chopra, Darren Dworkin, Michael Elrad, Joe Gutman, Jeff Hammes, Margaret Laws, Jeff Malehorn, Ted Meisel, Rafael Pascualy, Shawn Reigsecker, Jay Rosen, and Brenda Williams as well as our cofounder Andrew Swinand.

During the writing and editing process, we benefited enormously from the help of our literary agent Scott Hoffman and the staff of Folio literary agency. We are also grateful for the insights and advice offered by Michele Martin, head of the North Star Way imprint at Simon & Schuster, as well as our editor Kathryn Huck, senior editor at North Star Way. We would also like to thank Nancy Hancock, Naomi Lucks, and Leslie Tilley for their editorial assistance.

We are grateful to the many psychologists, neuroscientists, and philosophers who helped us review and fact check the manuscript. We owe a particular thanks to Dr. Susan Lape, who personally fact-checked every reference to the many ancient wisdom traditions. We would also like to thank Dr. Dan Gilbert, Dr. Greg Fricchione, Dr. James Miller, Stephen Mitchell, Dr. Jorge Moll, Dr. Josiah Ober, Matthieu Ricard, Dr. Robert Sapolsky, and Dr. Martin Seligman for their support and for reviewing our references to their work.

We owe the greatest thanks to our families, who not only offered insights and advice but also support and encouragement along the way. This book is dedicated to Eric's wife, Sharon, and Nate's wife, Kaley—two amazing women who have offered countless contributions to LIFE XT and to our lives. We're also grateful for the love and support of our children: Nate's daughter, Jorie; Eric's sons, Matthew and Alex, and his daughter, Elizabeth. Finally, we are deeply grateful for the guiding encouragement of our amazing parents: Eric's dad, Hugo, and stepmother, Louise; Nate's dad, Joe, and his mom, Margi.

Appendix 1: Habit Formation

Many of our day-to-day activities involve habit. For the most part, habits streamline the efficiency of our everyday life. They increase our productivity by making everyday tasks easier and quicker to complete. When you write an email, for example, a lifetime of habits kicks in. You don't have to relearn how to type or spell. Instead, your brain acts with extraordinary efficiency, relying on years of habituation and wired neural pathways to speedily complete the task. Scientists call this *automaticity*. Well-developed habits reduce the amount of both active brain processing power and motivation required to accomplish tasks. Habits, in other words, are the brain's way of acting with minimal conscious effort and maximum efficiency.

As a consequence, much of what we achieve in life is a direct result of having formed good habits. This is especially true when integrating the LIFE XT practices into our day-to-day lives, which are designed to help you create new, more efficient habits that result in a more optimal state of wellbeing.

But how do habits work? Consider an everyday habit: checking our smartphone. Most of us have experienced this almost irresistible desire to check our phone, whether it's for texts, emails, or NFL scores, or Facebook, Instagram, or Twitter. For some, this habit kicks in the moment we wake up. For others, it arises during moments of boredom. And for others, it surfaces during some of the most inappropriate moments: on a date, in a dark movie theater, or in the middle of a wedding ceremony.

Recent scientific research tells us that this habit, like all our habits, emerges from a small area of the brain called the basal ganglia, located just above the brain stem. Scientists further theorize that all of our habits run along a loop of cue, routine, and reward:[1]

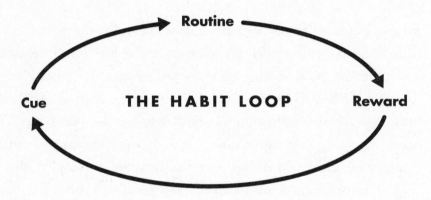

The cue could be anything—a sound, a sight, a thought, or a feeling. When you perceive it, the cue activates the habit. In the smartphone example, the notification sound activates the loop: You hear the ring or chime of your phone (the cue), which leads you to pull it out of your purse or pocket and check it (the routine). Then comes the reward—that almost instantaneous burst of dopamine-induced pleasure that you experience as you open the email, read the text, or glance at the game score. The more we travel this loop of habit, the more ingrained these neurologically driven routines become, and the more difficult it is to resist glancing down at our phones.

What's going on? The short burst of pleasure that we experience as the reward draws us into this loop. The irony, of course, is that the experience of pleasure never lasts, and at times it can be almost imperceptible. The rush disappears. The buzz goes away. The high ends, usually within seconds. As Sam Harris puts it, pleasures "begin to subside the instant they arise, only to be replaced by fresh desires or feelings of discomfort."[2] So goes the endless, often irrational dance of habit: We seek out momentary pleasure as a way to satisfy discomfort. After a few seconds the discomfort returns (often more intensely), and we begin seeking out the next momentary pleasure.

Just as good habits have the power to help us achieve greatness, bad habits have the potential to adversely shape our lives. Habits like excessive TV watching, work, eating, and drug abuse can keep us caught in negative patterns of stress, distraction, and anxiety. These habits of the mind and body silently seduce us into behaviors that result in the very opposite of wellbeing and happiness.

Making the Shift

How do we shift these deep-seated habits? It's not practical to change the cues, the first part of the loop. If you're addicted to your phone, your email, or other digital distractions, it's impractical to destroy your devices so that they never tempt you. If you have a tendency to react with anger during difficult conversations, you can't rid the world of disagreement or conflict. The cues that cause us to react are an inescapable part of life.

However, we can change the routine. Charles Duhigg calls this *the golden rule of habit:* "To change a habit, you must keep the old cue, and deliver the old reward, but insert a new routine."[3] Throughout LIFE XT, you engage in this process of shifting from old routines that generate stress, worry, and irritation to new, more productive routines. When we create these new habits, we not only introduce more positive behaviors into our lives. We also activate and reinforce new neural connections in our brain.

As you embark on this process, there are two critical steps to establishing new routines: First, setting intentions and, second, taking action. Here are a few tips to help you with both of these steps.

Stage 1: Setting Intentions

Begin by setting an intention to develop a new habit or change an existing habit.

- *Marshal your willpower carefully.* Willpower is the engine that drives habit change. It compels us to action. Yet it is also a finite resource. So be wary of trying to change too many habits at once. We simply don't have sufficient willpower. As a result, it is best to be strategic in your approach to habit change, layering on new habits one by one. It's also worth considering that, for most of us, the power of will is greater at the beginning of the day. This is perhaps why so many LIFE XT participants have found that it is best to build the Train practices into their morning routine.

- *Make a 100 percent commitment.* Research on habit confirms that the strength of commitment plays an essential role in the successful adoption of new habits. The best way to form a new habit is to make a 100 percent commitment to weave these practices into your day. In fact, we have found that it's actually much more difficult to make a 99 percent commitment. That 1 percent introduces choice and indecision into the equation. If you're 99 percent committed to walking every day, the 1 percent opens the possibility of not walking on any given day and can create unnecessary inner turmoil: *Maybe today should be my day off* or *I'll skip just this once.* A 100 percent commitment silences the indecision: *I'm going to walk today. I have made a commitment. There's no room for debate.*

Stage 2: Taking Action

Once you have marshaled your willpower and set an intention to develop or change a habit, the next step is to put this change in motion.

- *Identify the cues.* BJ Fogg describes the importance of identifying the kinds of behavioral triggers (cues) that you will use to develop a new habit routine and recommends using the following construct: "After (cue) _____, I will _____."[4] For example, *After I brush my teeth in the morning, I will meditate,* or *After I walk out the door, I will Notice-Shift-Rewire to compassion.*

- *Start slowly and small.* Setting yourself up for success is a key step, and we advise that you always establish modest, measurable, and realistic goals that you intuitively know are achievable. Doing so enables you to focus all your willpower on the goals you most wish to achieve. Start small. Celebrate success. Build slowly.

- *Be consistent and never miss a day.* This is how we actualize our 100 percent commitment to a new habit. Finding a consistent time and place to practice is also key. Try to meditate at the same time each day in the same place. Exercise on similar days of the week or at similar times. The more you achieve consistency, the more you will begin experiencing the efficiency-boosting benefits of habit.

- *Give it time.* The self-sustaining efficiency of habit takes time to develop—anywhere from 18 to 250 days.[5] Written in the third century BCE, the Dhammapada echoes the idea that forming new habits can take time: "Little by little a person

becomes evil, as a water pot is filled by drops of water . . .
Little by little a person becomes good, as a water pot is filled
by drops of water."[6] New neural connections take time to develop, but each little bit, "each drop," causes neurons to fire
and wire together. Sustaining the habit will get easier with
each passing drop.

- *Track your progress.* Use the LIFE XT dashboard or some
  other tracking tool to monitor your progress. The daily act of
  entering your practice data and seeing your progress toward
  your goal, your streaks of consistent practice, and other measures of success will serve as a source of positive reinforce-
  ment.

- *Develop a support system.* Having a training partner will help
  you stay motivated and offer an external source of accountability. You can support each other by checking in each week
  about whether you hit your practice goals.

- *Celebrate victory and reward yourself.* As you now know, habits
  require reward. The technique that we advise is simple: savor.
  At the end of each meditation, savor the experience of feeling more grounded, relaxed, and at ease. When you move,
  savor the clarity of mind and endorphin-driven elevation in
  mood. Put your hands in the air, smile, and give yourself some
  positive affirmation. Try it now and see how it feels. Savoring these moments will help you remember the powerful reward offered by these life habits—a reward that goes beyond
  momentary pleasure and cultivates a more enduring state of
  wellbeing.

- *Adopt a growth mind-set.* If you stumble, tell yourself *I am better than this.* Do not start the negative cycle of a self-defeating
  narrative such as *I am bad.*

It's easy to get overwhelmed by all these strategies and scientific details of habit formation. The important thing to remember is that your habits will change. Building new, more productive habits requires identifying a cue, making a 100 percent commitment, staying consistent in your practice, and rewarding yourself for success.

Habit formation is the most essential ingredient in training the skill of wellbeing—one that runs through all of LIFE XT. It's the way that we shift out of a lifetime of behaviors that keeps us tethered to our default happiness set point. By forming lifelong habits of wellbeing, we turn the experience of happiness into an efficient everyday state. We no longer need to work so hard to shift our experience of life. This shift becomes automatic.

Appendix 2: The Triune Brain

One of the key ideas of the chapter on the happiness set point is that we are running modern software on prehistoric hardware. This is what creates anxiety, vigilance, and the negativity bias in the brain that leads to suffering. But it is also a product of the evolution and underlying structure of the human brain. In the 1950s, neurologist Paul D. MacLean proposed a model called the triune brain that illustrates this paradoxical structure.[1] In this model, the brain is seen as a complex fusion of old and new: the reptilian brain, the paleomammalian brain, and the neomammalian brain.

The Reptilian Brain

Sitting at the base of the human brain and at the top of the spinal cord is the reptilian brain, the most primitive region of the brain. Key sections of the reptilian brain include the brain stem, medulla, pons, and cerebellum. Because this region of the brain was the first to develop, it is also the most primitive. It functions primarily as a kind of input/output mechanism of the brain: relaying all information from the body to the higher brain regions.[2] The reptilian brain also controls basic bodily functions like respiration, heart rate, and balance. It also sends important messages to the higher brain regions. When you are hungry or sexually aroused, the brain stem activates other regions of the brain.[3]

The Paleomammalian Brain

The second brain region to evolve—the paleomammalian or limbic region—lies just above the brain stem, deep inside the brain. This brain region consists of the hypothalamus, amygdala, and hippocampus. If we had only the reptilian brain to work with, our lives would be solitary and centered on little more than survival. However, while it is also involved in survival functions, the limbic part of the brain also plays a key role in higher-level functions such as motivation, emotion, and relationships with others. John Cacioppo explains, "With the advent of the paleomammalian (or emotional) brain in more advanced species, the social bonds between individuals began to become more complex and adaptable."[4]

If you just had these first two brain regions, you might live the life of a rat, a cat, or a dog.[5] You would experience primitive survival instincts and feel basic emotions, as well as a strong desire to attach to others. But you would not be reading this book. You would not be thinking about how to improve your life because you would have no sense of *you*—no idea of yourself as something separate.

The Neomammalian Brain

Enter the final region of the brain: the neomammalian brain, or cortex. This is the outermost layer of the brain and the final product of evolution. It first arose in primates but reached its apotheosis in the human brain. It's where mental maps, concepts, insights, and ideas arise. Cacioppo explains that this region of the brain "controls higher-order processes such as thinking, reasoning, language, problem solving, emotional regulation, and self-control."[6]

This final part of the brain gives us the tools we need to train the skill of wellbeing—to begin to understand and integrate the conflicting messages of the reptilian and paleomammalian brains. When the brain stem yells *Snake!* the prefrontal region of the cortex can take a step back, evaluate the situation, and help us determine whether what we thought was a snake might actually just be an old rope lying on the trail.

What LIFE XT calls the set point forces—judgment, attachment, and resistance—emanate from all three of these brain regions. As you move up through the layers of the triune brain, these basic functions are represented again and again in increasingly abstract ways. In the limbic region, we begin to make evaluations of our situation (judgment), move toward (attach), and move away (resist). At this level of the brain, these are just impulses. In the cortex, however, they are represented once more in a more complex form. They become concepts, thoughts, and ideas. The cortex allows us to make these impulses meaningful and to make long-term decisions about what is in our best interest.[7] The limbic brain might move us toward the ice cream cone. The cortex allows us to consider whether it might be better to eat dinner first or have a bowl of fruit instead.

This is good news. This more sophisticated part of the brain can also make it more challenging to simply "be happy." The advanced capacities of the cortex allow us to think. Yet, as Daniel Siegel explains, "the burden is that at times these new capacities allow us to think too much."[8] When not properly trained and integrated, our capacity to think frequently sows the seeds of worry, resentment, and unease.

Left Brain, Right Brain

In recent times, the terms *left brain* and *right brain* have become a bit of a cultural cliché. Creative people are called right brain, while more logical and rational people are seen as left brain. The reality is that both sides of the brain play an essential role in shaping our experience. Yet there are important differences between them.

The now-famous story of neuroanatomist Jill Bolte Taylor offers a window into what happens when one side of the brain stops functioning properly. In 1996, Taylor had a stroke in left side of her brain. With her left hemisphere off-line, she reported an almost mystical experience:

> My left hemisphere brain chatter went totally silent. Just like someone took a remote control and pushed the mute button and—total silence. And at first I was shocked to find myself inside of a silent mind. But then I was immediately captivated by the magnificence of energy around me. And because I could no longer identify the boundaries of my body, I felt enormous and expansive. I felt at one with all the energy that was, and it was beautiful there.[9]

Of course, Taylor's experience wasn't completely blissful. She also experienced the loss of the essential functions of her left hemisphere: She could no longer talk or even think in a clear, linear way. Amazingly, though, her left hemisphere recovered.

Taylor's experience points to the differences between these two sides of the brain. The left hemisphere helps us engage in linguistic, linear, and logical thinking. The right hemisphere, by contrast, helps us process more holistic, nonverbal forms of information.[10] It processes visual and auditory information, bodily sensations, and spontaneous emotional experiences. It's what gave Taylor the capacity to feel at one with the universe and the present moment.

Like the vertical structures of the triune brain, the coordinated functioning of these horizontal structures of the right brain and the left brain help determine our wellbeing. Depression, anxiety, and other states of psychological distress often correspond to a right-side imbalance.[11] By using the practices of LIFE XT to train the skill of attention, however, we create a more integrated brain state by shifting the patterns of activation to the left side of the brain. Siegel explains, "mindfulness appears to lead toward an approach state, with a left sided shift in frontal activity."[12]

From a scientific perspective, the LIFE XT program is designed to help you integrate these underlying structures of the brain—to create new neural connections between the three vertical and two horizontal regions of the brain. The goal is to integrate the brain in ways that reduce suffering, promote wellbeing, and enable you to achieve a felt sense of aliveness (being) and bring your greatest possible contribution to the world (doing).

Bibliography

For Further Reading

We encourage you to continue exploring the wisdom, science, and practice of Life Cross Training. If you are interested in delving deeper into the nine practices, here are the books on each practice that have had the most profound impact on our lives.

Meditation

Bhante Henepola Gunaratana. *Mindfulness in Plain English.* Updated and expanded ed. Somerville, MA: Wisdom Publications, 2002.

Bokar Rinpoche. *Meditation: Advice to Beginners,* 2nd ed. San Francisco: ClearPoint Press, 1999.

Easwaran, Eknath. *Meditation.* Tomales, CA: Nilgiri Press, 1993.

———. *Conquest of the Mind.* Tomales, CA: Nilgiri Press, 2010.

Hanh, Thich Nhat. *The Miracle of Mindfulness.* Boston: Beacon Press, 1976.

Kabat-Zinn, Jon. *Coming to Our Senses.* New York: Hyperion, 2005.

———. *Wherever You Go, There You Are.* New York: Hyperion, 2004.

Kornfield, Jack. *A Path with Heart.* New York: Bantam, 1993.

Mipham, Sakyong. *Turning the Mind into an Ally.* New York: Riverhead Books, 2003.

Ricard, Matthieu. *Why Meditate?* New York: Hay House, 2010.

Salzberg, Sharon. *Real Happiness.* New York: Workman Publishing Company, 2011.

Suzuki, Shunryu. *Zen Mind, Beginner's Mind.* Boston: Weatherhill, 2006.

Wallace, B. Alan. *The Attention Revolution: Unlocking the Power of the Focused Mind.* Somerville, MA: Wisdom Publications, 2006.

Yongey Mingyur Rinpoche and Eric Swanson. *The Joy of Living: Unlocking the Secret and Science of Happiness.* New York: Harmony Books, 2007.

Meditation

Davidson, Richard. *The Emotional Life of Your Brain.* New York: Hudson Street Books, 2012.

Farb, Norman A. S., et al. "Attending to the Present: Mindfulness Meditation Reveals Distinct Neural Modes of Self-Reference." *Social Cognitive and Affective Neuroscience* 2, no. 4 (2007): 313–22.

Goleman, Daniel. *Destructive Emotions: How Can We Overcome Them?* New York: Bantam Books, 2003.

Siegel, Daniel. *The Mindful Brain.* New York: Norton, 2007.

Movement

Broad, William J. *The Science of Yoga.* New York: Simon & Schuster, 2012.

Lyubomirsky, Sonja. *The How of Happiness.* New York: Penguin Press, 2008.

Ratey, John J. *Spark: The Revolutionary New Science of Exercise and the Brain.* New York: Little, Brown, 2008.

Saunders, Travis. "Can Sitting Too Much Kill You?" *Scientific American,* January 2011.

Thoreau, Henry David. "Walking," in *The Portable Thoreau.* New York: Penguin, 1975.

Inquiry

Katie, Byron. *Loving What Is.* New York: Harmony Books, 2002.

———. *A Thousand Names for Joy.* New York: Harmony Books, 2007.

Lao-tzu. *Tao Te Ching.* Translated by Stephen Mitchell. New York: Harper Perennial, 1988.

Miller, James. *Examined Lives.* New York: Farrar, Straus, and Giroux, 2011.

Plato. "The Apology." In *Plato's Apology, Crito, and Phaedo*. Translated by Henry Cary. Philadelphia: David McKay Publisher, 1897.

Sapolsky, Robert. *Why Zebras Don't Get Ulcers*. New York: Holt Paperbacks, 2004.

Seligman, Martin E. P. *Learned Optimism*. New York: Vintage, 2006.

Presence

Hanh, Thich Nhat. *The Miricle of Mindfulness*. Boston: Beacon Press, 1976.

Kabat-Zinn, Jon. *Coming to Our Senses*. New York: Hyperion, 2005.

Thoreau, Henry David. "Walden," in *The Portable Thoreau*. New York: Penguin, 1947.

Gratitude

Emmons, Robert A., and Michael E. McCullough. "Counting Blessings Versus Burdens." *Journal of Personality and Social Psychology* 84, no. 2 (2003): 377–89.

Hanson, Rick. *Buddha's Brain*. Oakland: New Harbinger Publications, 2009.

Lyubomirsky, Sonja. *The How of Happiness*. New York: Penguin Press, 2008.

Seligman, Martin E. P. *Authentic Happiness*. New York: Free Press, 2002.

Compassion

Buddha. *The Dhammapada*. Translated by Eknath Easwaran. Tomales, CA: Nilgiri Press, 2007.

Davidson, Richard. *The Emotional Life of Your Brain*. New York: Hudson Street Books, 2012.

Easwaran, Eknath. *Gandhi: The Man*. Tomales, CA: Nilgiri Press, 1997.

Lao-tzu. *Tao Te Ching*. Translated by Stephen Mitchell. New York: Harper Perennial, 1988.

Yongey Mingyur Rinpoche and Eric Swanson. *The Joy of Living: Unlocking the Secret and Science of Happiness*. New York: Harmony Books, 2007.

Engagement

Chuang Tzu. *The Inner Chapters*. Translated by David Hinton. New York: Counterpoint, 1998.

Csikszentmihalyi, Mihaly. *Flow: The Psychology of Optimal Experience*. New York: Harper Perennial, 1990.

Loehr, Jim, and Tony Schwartz. *The Power of Full Engagement*. New York: Free Press, 2003.

Seligman, Martin E. P. *Authentic Happiness*. New York: Free Press, 2002.

Relationships

Aristotle. *The Nicomachean Ethics*. New York: Penguin, 2004.

Cacioppo, John T., and William Patrick. *Loneliness*. New York: Norton, 2008.

Krakauer, Jon. *Into the Wild*. New York: Anchor, 1997.

Seligman, Martin E. P. *Flourish*. New York: Free Press, 2011.

Taylor, Jill Bolte. *My Stroke of Insight*. New York: Plume, 2009.

Contribution

Fox, Michael J. *Lucky Man*. New York: Hyperion, 2002.

McClelland, David, and Carol Kirshnit. "The Effect of Motivational Arousal Through Films on Salivary Immunoglobulin A." *Psychology and Health* 2, no. 1 (1988): 31–52.

Seligman, Martin E. P. *Flourish*. New York: Free Press, 2011.

Notes

The Open Secret

1 https://www.apa.org/news/press/releases/stress/2012/full-report
.pdf.

2 Paul Rosch, "Job Stress: America's Leading Adult Health Problem,"
USA Magazine, May 1991. See also "American Academy of Family
Physicians Survey," *US News and World Report,* December 11, 1995.

3 Filix Richter, "Americans Use Electronic Media 11+ Hours a Day,"
Statistica, March 13, 2015; Joanna Stern, "Cell Phone Users Check
Phones 150x Day," *ABC News,* May 29, 2013.

4 Matthew A. Killingsworth and Daniel T. Gilbert, "A Wandering
Mind Is an Unhappy Mind," *Science* 330, no. 6006 (2010), 111.

5 We hear words like *happiness* all the time, and it's easy to get
thrown off by their close association with short bursts of pleasure: eating ice cream, watching television, or buying that new
car you've always wanted. This is not the happiness that we write
about. Rather, *Start Here* uses the words *wellbeing* and *happiness* to
describe something deeper: the moment-to-moment experience
of a life well lived. In the context of *Start Here, happiness* and *wellbeing* describe the more profound lasting experience of navigating
life's challenges with an underlying sense of peace and purpose.

6 P90X or "Power 90 Extreme" is a popular home exercise program
based on the idea of cross training and muscle confusion.

Understanding Our Set Point

1 Robert Sapolsky, *Why Zebras Don't Get Ulcers* (New York: Holt Paperbacks, 2004).

2 Ibid., 4.

3 Paul Rozin, "Negativity Bias, Negativity Dominace, and Cognition," *Personality and Social Psychology Review* 5, no. 4 (2001).

4 Rick Hanson, *Buddha's Brain* (Oakland: New Harbinger Publications, 2009), 41.

5 Ibid., 43–44.

6 P. Brickman, "Lottery Winners and Accident Victims: Is Happiness Relative?" *Journal of Personality and Social Psychology* 36, no. 8 (1978).

7 Lao-tzu, *Tao Te Ching*, trans. Stephen Mitchell (New York: Harper Perennial, 1988).

8 Jill Bolte Taylor, *My Stroke of Insight* (New York: Plume, 2009), 2.

9 *World Scripture: A Comparative Anthology of Sacred Texts*, ed. Andrew Wilson (New York: International Religious Foundation, dist. Paragon House, 1991), 658.

10 Richard Davidson, *The Emotional Life of Your Brain* (New York: Hudson Street Press, 2012), 40.

11 Cacioppo et al., *Foundations in Social Neuroscience*, 1049.

12 Davidson, *The Emotional Life of Your Brain*, 40.

13 We are grateful to Dr. Jeanne Talbot for her insights and for contributing this passage on the nature of "experiential avoidance."

Stage 1: Train

1 Richard Davidson, *The Emotional Life of Your Brain* (New York: Hudson Street Press, 2012), 179.

2 Years later, Eric ended up having a similar experience while attending a meditation retreat in the same system of vipassana.

3 Davidson, *The Emotional Life of Your Brain*, 182.

4 Ibid., 183.

5 Marta Tarbell, "Be Happy Like a Monk," *Telluride Watch*, March 26, 2007.

6 Aristotle, *The Nicomachean Ethics* (New York: Penguin, 2004), 31.

7 William James, "Habit," in *The Writings of William James*, ed. John McDermott (Chicago: University of Chicago Press, 1977), 12.

8 Ibid., 10.

9 William James, *The Principles of Psychology* (New York: Henry Holt, 1890), 402.

10 Norman Doidge, *The Brain That Changes Itself* (New York: Penguin Books, 2007), xviii.

11 Davidson, *The Emotional Life of Your Brain*, 161.

12 Doidge, *The Brain That Changes Itself*, 63.

13 Donald O. Hebb, *The Organization of Behavior: A Neuropsychological Theory* (New York: Wiley, 1949).

14 Jill Bolte Taylor, *My Stroke of Insight* (New York: Plume, 2009), 177.

Practice 1: Meditation

1 "Katy Perry: Meditation Brings More Creativity and Positive Energy," *MindBodyGreen*, October 23, 2012. http://www.mindbodygreen .com/0-6583/Katy-Perry-Meditation-Brings-More-Creativity -Positive-Energy.html.

2 Oprah Winfrey, "What Oprah Knows for Sure About Finding the Fullest Expression of Yourself," *The Oprah Magazine*, February 2012; http://www.oprah.com/health/Oprah-on-Stillness-and -Meditation-Oprah-Visits-Fairfield-Iowa.

3 Richard Davidson, *The Emotional Life of Your Brain* (New York: Hudson Street Press, 2012), 183.

4 Alyssa Roenigk, "Lotus Pose on Two," *ESPN The Magazine*, August 23, 2013.

5 Matthieu Ricard, personal website, http://www.matthieuricard .org/en/index.php/about/.

6 Daniel Goleman, *Destructive Emotions: How Can We Overcome Them?* (New York: Bantam Books, 2003), 9.

7 Ibid., 12.

8 Ibid., 15.

9 Ibid.

10 Matthieu Ricard, Antoine Lutz, and Richard J. Davidson, "Neuroscience Reveals the Secrets of Meditation's Benefits," *Scientific American*, November 1, 2014; http://www.scientificamerican.com /article/neuroscience-reveals-the-secrets-of-meditation-s-bene fits/.

11 We are grateful to Matthieu Ricard for providing us with this passage on the nature of presence.

12 *World Scripture: A Comparative Anthology of Sacred Texts*, ed. Andrew Wilson (New York: International Religious Foundation, dist. Paragon House, 1991), 603.

13 Buddha, *The Dhammapada*, trans. Eknath Easwaran (Tomales, CA: Nilgiri Press, 2007), 115.

14 Pierre Hadot, *Philosophy as a Way of Life* trans. Michael Chase (Malden, MA: Blackwell Publishing, 1995), 59.

15 Marcus Aurelius, *Meditations*, 9:32, quote taken from John Sellars, *The Art of Living.* (New York: Bloomberg Academic, 2003), 150.

16 Davidson, *The Emotional Life of Your Brain*, 200.

17 Ibid., 202–3.

18 Ibid., 203.

19 Ibid., 204.

20 Ibid.

21 J. A. Brefczynski-Lewis et al., "Neural Correlates of Attentional Expertise in Long-Term Meditation Practitioners," *Proceedings of the National Academy of Sciences* 104, no. 27 (2007).

22 Norman A. Farb et al., "Attending to the Present: Mindfulness Meditation Reveals Distinct Neural Modes of Self-Reference," *Social Cognitive and Affective Neuroscience* 2, no. 4 (2007).

23 David W. Orme-Johnson et al., "Neuroimaging of Meditation's Effect on Brain Reactivity to Pain," *Neuroreport* 17, no. 12 (2006).

24 Sara W. Lazar et al., "Meditation Experience Is Associated with Increased Cortical Thickness," *Neuroreport* 16, no. 17 (2005).

25 Matthieu Ricard, *Why Meditate?* (New York: Hay House, 2010), 14.

26 Richard Davidson et al., "Alterations in Brain and Immune Function Produced by Mindfulness Meditation," *Psychosomatic Medicine* 65, no. 4 (2003): 565.

27 Fred Travis et al., "Effects of Transcendental Meditation Practice on Brain Functioning and Stress Reactivity in College Students," *International Journal of Psychophysiology* 71, no. 2 (2008).

28 Shunryu Suzuki, *Zen Mind, Beginner's Mind* (Boston: Shambhala, 2006), 26.

29 Ricard, *Why Meditate?*, 71.

30 Suzuki, *Zen Mind, Beginner's Mind*, 34.

31 While the words *present moment* and *nonjudgmental* are widely used as instructional cues for how to meditate, some scholars of Buddhism argue that these terms do not offer an accurate account of the actual practice of meditation. Georges Dreyfus, for example, argues that classical accounts describe the essence of meditation as building the "capacity to hold its object and thus allow for sustained attention." This object could be something from the past. Further, meditation could involve judgments between right and wrong, a capacity of dis-

cernment that is distinct from the impulsive judgments that arise in nonmeditative states. Dreyfus claims that the fact that meditation can involve thoughts about past and future as well as judgments shows that the widely held description of meditation as present and nonjudgmental overlooks some of the key features of meditation practice. See Georges Dreyfus, "Is Mindfulness Present-Centered and Non-Judgmental? A Discussion of the Cognitive Dimensions of Mindfulness," *Contemporary Buddhism* 12, no. 1 (2011).

32 We are grateful to David Chernikoff for his insight and teachings on this practice of open awareness meditation.

33 Joseph Goldstein and Jack Kornfield, *Seeking the Heart of Wisdom* (Boston: Shambhala Classics, 1987), 30–37.

34 Jon Kabat-Zinn, *Coming to Our Senses* (New York: Hyperion, 2005), 23.

35 Email correspondence with Matthieu Ricard, August 7, 2013.

36 Yongey Mingyur Rinpoche and Eric Swanson, *The Joy of Living: Unlocking the Secret and Science of Happiness.* (New York: Harmony Books, 2007), 12–13.

37 Ibid., 21–22.

Practice 2: Movement

1 Henry David Thoreau, "Walking," in *The Portable Thoreau* (New York: Penguin, 1975), 597.

2 Friedrich Nietzsche, *Twilight of the Idols* (Indianapolis: Hackett Publishing, 1997), 10.

3 Ibid.

4 Christopher Shields, "Aristotle," *The Stanford Encyclopedia of Philosophy* (Spring 2014 Edition), ed. Edward N. Zalta; http://plato.stanford.edu/archives/spr2014/entries/aristotle/. We are grateful to Susan Lape for this reference.

5 Diogenes Laertius, *Lives of Eminent Philosophers*, Book 7, trans. R. D. Hicks (Boston: Loeb Classical Library, Harvard University Press, 1925), 4; http://www.perseus.tufts.edu/hopper/text?doc=Perseus %3Atext%3A1999.01.0258%3Abook%3D7%3Achapter%3D1. We are grateful to Susan Lape for steering us toward this important text.

6 William J. Broad, *The Science of Yoga* (New York: Simon & Schuster 2012), 9.

7 Ibid., 56.

8 Ibid., 57.

9 Ibid., 100.

10 Manoj K. Bhasin et al., "Relaxation Response Induces Temporal Transcriptome Changes in Energy Metabolism, Insulin Secretion and Inflammatory Pathways," *PLOS ONE,* May 1, 2013; DOI: 10.1371/journal.pone.0062817.

11 John J. Ratey, *Spark: The Revolutionary New Science of Exercise and the Brain* (New York: Little, Brown, 2008), 53.

12 Ibid., 54.

13 Ibid., 83.

14 Ibid., 71.

15 Ibid., 122.

16 Ibid., 235–36.

17 Ibid., 232.

18 Alice Park, "Sitting Is Killing You," *Time*, September 2, 2014; http://time.com/sitting.

19 P. T. Katzmarzyk et al., "Sitting Time and Mortality from All Causes, Cardiovascular Disease, and Cancer," *Medicine and Science in Sports and Exercise* 41, no. 5 (2009).

20 Travis Saunders, "Can Sitting Too Much Kill You?," *Scientific American,* January (2011).

21 Ibid.

22 Thoreau, "Walking," 597.

Practice 3: Inquiry

1 Allison Adato, "How a Self-Help Guru Is Born," *Los Angeles Times*, November 24, 2002.

2 Ibid.

3 Byron Katie, *A Thousand Names for Joy* (New York: Harmony Books, 2007), 197.

4 Ibid., 86.

5 Adato, "How a Self-Help Guru Is Born."

6 Byron Katie, TheWork.com, http://www.thework.com.

7 Socrates, "Apology," in *Four Texts on Socrates*, trans. with notes by Thomas G. West and Grace Starry West (Ithaca: Cornell University Press, 1984), 83.

8 We are grateful to James Miller for reviewing our discussion of his work. See James Miller, *Examined Lives* (New York: Farrar, Straus, and Giroux, 2011), 21.

9 Miller, *Examined Lives*, 23.

10 We are grateful for Stanford University professor Josiah Ober's comments on our description of Socrates.

11 Socrates, "Apology," 71.

12 Plato, "The Apology," in *Plato's Apology, Crito, and Phaedo*, trans. Henry Cary (Philadelphia: David McKay Publisher, 1897), 19.

13 Byron Katie, *Loving What Is* (New York: Harmony Books, 2002), viii.

14 William Shakespeare, *Hamlet* (London: William Heinemann, 1904), 50.

15 Katja Vogt, "Ancient Skepticism," *The Stanford Encyclopedia of Philosophy* (Summer 2015 Edition), ed. Edward N. Zalta; http://plato.stanford.edu/archives/sum2015/entries/skepticism-ancient. We are grateful to Susan Lape for helping us see the parallels between the Inquiry practice and ancient skepticism.

16 Shunryu Suzuki, *Zen Mind, Beginner's Mind* (Boston: Shambhala, 2006), 21–22.

17 We are grateful to Stephen Mitchell, who shared this with us in an email conversation on October 7, 2015.

18 Khenpo Tsültrim Gyamtso Rinpoche, *Progressive Stages of Meditation on Emptiness* (Onemana: Zhyisil Chokyi Ghatsal Publications, 2000), 57.

19 Andrew C. Butler et al., "The Empirical Status of Cognitive-Behavioral Therapy: A Review of Meta-Analyses," *Clinical Psychology Review* 26 (2006).

20 Albert Ellis and Windy Dryden, *The Practice of Rational Emotive Behavior Therapy* (New York: Springer Publishing Company, 2007), 2.

21 Ibid., 16.

22 Martin E. P. Seligman, *Learned Optimism* (New York: Vintage, 2006), 89–90.

23 For more resources and information on "The Work," go to www.TheWork.com.

Stages 2 and 3: Be and Do

1 Bill Russell and Taylor Branch, *Second Wind: The Memoirs of an Opinionated Man* (New York: Random Houses, 1979), 155–57.

2 Ibid., 155.

3 Ibid., 156.

4 Ibid.

5 Ibid.

6 Ibid., 157.

7 Ibid.

8 Conversation with John Cacioppo on June 19, 2013.

9 Henry David Thoreau, "Walking," in *The Portable Thoreau* (New York: Penguin, 1975), 343.

10 Ibid.

11 Vladimir Antonov, *Classics of Spiritual Philosophy and the Present* (Essex: New Atlanteans, 2009), 81.

12 Plato, "The Apology," in *Plato's Apology, Crito, and Phaedo*, trans. Henry Cary (Philadelphia: David McKay Publisher, 1897), 31a.

Notice-Shift-Rewire

1 Elizabeth Gilbert, *Eat, Pray, Love* (New York: Penguin Books, 2007), 41.

2 Byron Katie, "Unshakeable Inner Peace," TheWork.com. http://www.byronkatie.com/2014/12/unshakeable-inner-peace.

3 Romeo Vitelli, "Letting Your Mind Wander," *Psychology Today*, April 15, 2013; https://www.psychologytoday.com/blog/media -spotlight/201304/letting-your-mind-wander.

4 Matthew A. Killingsworth and Daniel T. Gilbert, "A Wandering Mind Is an Unhappy Mind," *Science* 330, no. 6006 (2010).

5. Ibid.

6 Steve Bradt, "Wandering Mind Not a Happy Mind," *Harvard Gazette*, November 11, 2010; http://news.harvard.edu/gazette/story /2010/11/wandering-mind-not-a-happy-mind/.

7 We are grateful to Dan Gilbert for reviewing our description of his work.

8 Daniel J. Siegel, *The Mindful Brain* (New York: Norton, 2007), 178.

9 Donald O. Hebb, *The Organization of Behavior: A Neuropsychological Theory* (New York: Wiley, 1949), 62.

10 Daniel J. Siegel, *Mindsight: The New Science of Personal Transformation* (New York: Bantam Books, 2010), 43.

11 Buddha, *The Dhammapada*, trans. Eknath Easwaran (Berkeley, CA: Nilgiri Press, 2007), 224.

12 Ibid.

13 Aristotle, *The Nicomachean Ethics* (New York: Penguin, 2004), 3: 1094a.

14 Ralph Waldo Emerson, "Fate," in *The Portable Emerson* (New York: Penguin, 1981), 361.

15 Eyal Ophir, Clifford Nass, and Anthony D. Wagner, "Cognitive Control in Media Multitaskers," *Proceedings of the National Academy of Sciences* 106, no. 37 (2009).

Practice 4: Presence

1 Michael Brown, *The Presence Process* (Vancouver, BC: Namaste Publishing, 2012), xxvii.

2 Jordan Gaines Lewis, "Why Does Time Fly as We Get Older?," *Scientific American*, December 18, 2013; http://blogs.scientific american.com/mind-guest-blog/why-does-time-fly-as-we-get -older.

3 John Dewey, *The Later Works of John Dewey*, volume 14 (Carbondale: Southern Illinois University Press, 2008), 131.

4 On the importance of the present moment in the Stoic tradition, see Pierre Hadot, *Philosophy as a Way of Life*, trans. Michael Chase (Malden, MA: Blackwell Publishing, 1995), 227; Marcus Aurelius, *Meditations* (New York: Penguin Classics, 1964), 6–9; Seneca, *On Benefits* (Chicago: University of Chicago Press, 2010), 7, 2, 4–5. We are grateful to Susan Lape for identifying these additional resources.

5 Hadot, *Philosophy as a Way of Life*.

6 Ibid., 224. See also Epicurus, *Vatican Sayings*, 14; http://www.epi curus.net/en/vatican.html.

7 Hadot, *Philosophy as a Way of Life*, 221.

8 We are grateful to Susan Lape for helping us discover that, while

quoted from Cicero's *On Ends*, the passage is actually Cicero's description of the Epicureans; Hadot, *Philosophy as a Way of Life,* 223.

9 Ibid., 227.

10 We are grateful to David Chernikoff for this insight.

11 Pema Chödrön, *Smile at Fear* (Boston, MA: Shambhala Audio, 2011); http://www.youtube.com/watch?v=CVRT-y2wTBY.

12 Ibid.

13 Here we are referencing the powerful line offered by the Buddha in the Dhammapada: "Little by little a person becomes evil, as a water pot is filled by drops of water . . . Little by little a person becomes good, as a water pot is filled by drops of water." See Buddha, *The Dhammapada*, trans. Eknath Easwaran (Tomales, CA: Nilgiri Press, 2007), 141.

Practice 5: Gratitude

1 Stephen J. Dubner, "What Is Stephen King Trying to Prove?," *New York Times Magazine*, August 13, 2000. We are grateful to Robert A. Emmons for directing us to this story. See Robert A. Emmons, *Thanks! How the New Science of Gratitude Can Make You Happier* (New York: Houghton Mifflin, 2007), 1.

2 Ibid.

3 Ibid.

4 Robert A. Emmons and Michael E. McCullough, "Counting Blessings Versus Burdens," *Journal of Personality and Social Psychology* 84, no. 2 (2003).

5 Sonja Lyubomirsky, *The How of Happiness* (New York: Penguin Press, 2008), 89.

6 Ram Dass, with Rameshwar Das, *Polishing the Mirror* (Boulder, CO: Sounds True Press, 2013).

7 *World Scripture: A Comparative Anthology of Sacred Texts*, ed. Andrew Wilson (New York: International Religious Foundation, dist. Paragon House, 1991), 556.

8 Ibid.

9 Ibid.

10 Margaret Graver, "Epictetus," *The Stanford Encyclopedia of Philosophy* (Spring 2013 Edition), ed. Edward N. Zalta; http://plato.stanford.edu/archives/spr2013/entries/epictetus/.

11 Epictetus, *The Discourse of Epictetus and Fragments* (New York: Digireads Publishing, 1895), cxxix.

12 Rick Hanson, *Buddha's Brain* (Oakland, CA: New Harbinger Publications, 2009), 68.

13 Leslie E. Sekerka and Barbara L. Fredrickson, "Working Positively Toward Transformative Cooperation," in *The Oxford Handbook of Positive Psychology and Work*, ed. P. Alex Linley, Susan Harrington, and Nicola Garcea (New York: Oxford University Press, 2013), 83.

14 Ibid.

15 Richard Davidson, *The Emotional Life of Your Brain* (New York: Hudson Street Press, 2012), 231.

16 Emmons and McCullough, "Counting Blessings Versus Burdens."

17 B. L. Fredrickson et al., "What Good Are Positive Emotions in Crises?," *Journal of Personality and Social Psychology* 84, no. 2 (2003).

18 Emmons, *Thanks!*, 33.

19 We are grateful to Sonja Lyubomirsky for this insight. See Lyubomirsky, *The How of Happiness*, 97.

Practice 6: Compassion

1 Eknath Easwaran, *Gandhi: The Man*, 3rd ed. (Tomales, CA: Nilgiri Press, 1997), 97.

2 Ibid.

3 Ibid.

4 Ibid., 56.

5 We are grateful to Priti Patel for this insight about compassion arising from the combination of empathy and love.

6 Buddha, *The Dhammapada*, trans. Eknath Easwaran (Tomales, CA: Nilgiri Press, 2007), 703.

7 Lao-tzu, *Tao Te Ching*, trans. Stephen Mitchell (New York: Harper Perennial, 1988), 49.

8 Easwaran, *Gandhi: The Man*, 126.

9 Richard Davidson, *The Emotional Life of Your Brain* (New York: Hudson Street Press, 2012), 218.

10 Ibid., 213.

11 Ibid., 222.

12 Helen Y. Weng et al., "Compassion Training Alters Altruism and Neural Responses to Suffering," *Psychological Science* 24, no. 7 (2013).

13 Ibid.

14 Ibid.

15 While most compassion meditations follow a similar structure, we are grateful to Jack Kornfield, one of the leading meditation teachers, for the specific phrasing of the compassion mantra. See Jack Kornfield, "Meditation on Lovingkindness," http://www.jackkornfield.com/2011/02/meditation-on-lovingkindness.

16 Ibid.

17 Ibid.

18 Yongey Mingyur Rinpoche and Eric Swanson. *The Joy of Living: Unlocking the Secret and Science of Happiness*. (New York: Harmony Books, 2007), 175.

A Prelude to Doing

1 Henry David Thoreau, "Walden," in *The Portable Thoreau* (New York: Penguin, 1947), 562.

Practice 7: Engagement

1 William James, *The Principles of Psychology* (New York: Henry Holt, 1890), 402.

2 Mihaly Csikszentmihalyi, *Flow: The Psychology of Optimal Experience* (New York: Harper Perennial, 1990), 4.

3 Mihaly Csikszentmihalyi, *Good Business: Leadership, Flow, and Making of Meaning*, (New York: Penguin, 2004), 75.

4 Andrew Cooper, *Playing in the Zone* (Boston: Shambhala, 1998), 34.

5 Paul Berliner, *Thinking in Jazz* (Chicago: University of Chicago Press, 1994), 392.

6 Csikszentmihalyi, *Good Business*, 70.

7 Csikszentmihalyi, *Flow: The Psychology of Optimal Experience*, 150.

8 Ibid.

9 Ibid.

10 Chuang Tzu, *The Inner Chapters*, trans. David Hinton (New York: Counterpoint, 1997), 39.

11 Ibid., 39–40.

12 Maurizio Viroli, *Niccolò's Smile* (New York: Farrar, Straus, and Giroux, 2000), 153.

13 Martin E. P. Seligman, *Authentic Happiness* (New York: Free Press, 2002), 116.

14 Csikszentmihalyi, *Flow: The Psychology of Optimal Experience*, 74.

15 Sonja Lyubomirsky, *The How of Happiness* (New York: Penguin Press, 2008), 182.

16 Seligman, *Authentic Happiness*, 117.

17 Ibid.

18 Jim Loehr and Tony Schwartz, *The Power of Full Engagement* (New York: Free Press, 2003), 36.

19 Ibid., 13.

20 Ibid., 33–34.

21 Susan Weinschenk, "Why We're All Addicted to Texts, Twitter, and Google," *Psychology Today*, September 11, 2012.

Practice 8: Relationships

1 Jon Krakauer, "Death of an Innocent: How Christopher McCandless Lost His Way in the Wilds," *Outside Magazine*, January 1993.

2 Jon Krakauer, *Into the Wild* (New York: Anchor Books, 1997), 169.

3 Aristotle, *The Nicomachean Ethics* (New York: Penguin, 2004), Book 8.1, 1155a5–6.

4 We are grateful for Josiah Ober's comments on our description of Aristotle's conception of friendship.

5 Aristotle, *The Nicomachean Ethics*, Book 8.1, 1155a29.

6 Ibid., 1156a30–1.

7 Jill Bolte Taylor, *My Stroke of Insight* (New York: Viking, 2008), 87.

8 Aristotle, *The Nicomachean Ethics*, Book 8.8, 1159a27–28.

9 Ibid., 1166b1.

10 Ibid., Book 8.9, 1166a1–2.

11 Ibid., Book 8.5 1157b34–35.

12 John T. Cacioppo and William Patrick, *Loneliness* (New York: Norton, 2008).

13 Ibid., 43.

14 Ibid.

15 Lydialyle Gibson, "The Nature of Loneliness," *University of Chicago Magazine*, November–December 2010.

16 Cacioppo and Patrick, *Loneliness*, 105.

17 We are grateful for John Cacioppo's insights during a February 2014 conversation.

18 Sonja Lyubomirsky, *The How of Happiness* (New York: Penguin Press, 2008), 138.

19 Ibid., 140.

20 Melissa A. Milkie, "Does the Amount of Time Mothers Spend with Children or Adolescents Matter?," *Journal of Marriage and Family*, no. 2 (2015).

Practice 9: Contribution

1 Michael J. Fox, *Lucky Man* (New York: Hyperion, 2002), 1.

2 Ibid., 5.

3 Ibid., 6.

4 Ibid.

5 *World Scripture: A Comparative Anthology of Sacred Texts*, ed. Andrew Wilson (New York: International Religious Foundation, dist. Paragon House, 1991), 688.

6 Ibid., 695.

7 Ibid., 697.

8 Ibid., 695.

9 David McClelland and Carol Kirshnit, "The Effect of Motivational Arousal Through Films on Salivary Immunoglobulin A," *Psychology and Health* 2, no. 1 (1988).

10 A 1997 study of cardiac patients found that those who spent time supporting other inpatient cardiac patients showed reduced levels of mortality as well as depression. See Gwynn Sullivan and Martin Sullivan, "Promoting Wellness in Cardiac Rehabilitation: Exploring the Role of Altruism," *Journal of Cardiovascular Nursing* 11, no. 3 (April 1997). For an excellent literature review of key re-

search in the area of contribution, see Stephen G. Post, "It's Good to Be Good: Science Says It's So," *Health Progress*, July–August (2009).

11 Similarly, a three-year study of women with multiple sclerosis arrived at a set of findings. Women with MS who helped other women with the disease showed increases in self-esteem and self-acceptance, see Carolyn Shwartz, "Teaching Coping Skills Enhances Quality of Life More than Peer Support," *Health Psychology* 18, no. 3 (1999).

12 For instance, a longitudinal study conducted by the Center for Health Care Evaluation at Stanford University also found volunteering or contributing to the lives of others to be associated with decreased mortality. See Alex Harris and Carl Thoresen, "Volunteering Is Associated with Delayed Mortality in Older People," *Journal of Health Psychology* 10, no. 6 (2005).

13 Jorge Moll et al., "Human Fronto-Mesolimbic Networks Guide Decisions About Charitable Donation," *Proceedings of the National Academy of Sciences* 103, no. 42 (2006).

14 Martin E. P. Seligman, *Flourish* (New York: Free Press, 2011), 12.

15 John Darley and Daniel Batson, "From Jerusalem to Jericho: A Study of Situational and Dispositional Variables in Helping Behavior," *Journal of Personality and Social Psychology* 27, no. 1 (1973).

16 Dalai Lama, "A Meeting of Faiths and Concern for the Outer and Inner Environment in Portland, Oregon," DalaiLama.com, May 10, 2013. http://www.dalailama.com/news/post/942-a -meeting-of-faiths-and-concern-for-the-outer-and-inner -environment-in-portland-oregon.

How to Practice Life Cross Training

1 "How Long Should You Stand—Rather than Sit—at Your Work Station?," University of Waterloo, https://uwaterloo.ca/kinesiology /how-long-should-you-stand-rather-sit-your-work-station.

2 Bryan Walsh, "The Dangers of Sitting at Work—and Standing," *Time,* April 13, 2011; http://healthland.time.com/2011/04/13 /the-dangers-of-sitting-at-work-and-standing/.

Bringing It All Together

1 Data drawn from a three-month study on the impact of LIFE XT on employees at a Chicago-based media agency.

2 T. S. Eliot, *Four Quartets* (New York: Houghton Mifflin, 2014), 220.

3 William James, *The Principles of Psychology* (New York: Henry Holt, 1890), 402.

4 Pema Chödrön, *Comfortable with Uncertainty* (Boston: Shambhala Press, 2002), 8.

5 Viktor Frankl, *Man's Search for Meaning* (Boston: Beacon Press, 2006), 75.

Appendix 1: Habit Foundation

1 Charles Duhigg, *The Power of Habit* (New York: Random House, 2012).

2 Sam Harris, *Waking Up* (New York: Simon & Schuster, 2014), 17.

3 Duhigg, *The Power of Habit,* 62.

4 BJ Fogg, "Forget Big Change, Start with a Tiny Habit," TedxTalks; https://www.youtube.com/watch?v=AdKUJxjn-R8.

5 Phillippa Lally et al., "How Are Habits Formed: Modelling Habit

Formation in the Real World," *European Journal of Social Psychology* 40, no. 6 (2010).

6 Buddha, *The Dhammapada*, trans. Eknath Easwaran (Tomales, CA: Nilgiri Press, 2007), 141.

Appendix 2: The Triune Brain

1 John T. Cacioppo and William Patrick, *Loneliness* (New York: Norton, 2008), 50.

2 We are grateful to John Cacioppo for this insight.

3 Daniel J. Siegel, *Mindsight: The New Science of Personal Transformation* (New York: Bantam Books, 2010), 16.

4 Cacioppo and Patrick, *Loneliness*, 126.

5 Siegel, *Mindsight: The New Science of Personal Transformation*, 17.

6 Cacioppo and Patrick, *Loneliness*, 50.

7 We are grateful to John Cacioppo for this insight.

8 Siegel, *Mindsight: The New Science of Personal Transformation*, 20.

9 Jill Bolte Taylor, "My Stroke of Insight," Ted.com, March 12, 2008.

10 Daniel J. Siegel, *The Mindful Brain* (New York: Norton, 2007), 46.

11 David Hecht, "Depression and the Hyperactive Right-Hemisphere," *Neuroscience Research* 68, no. 2 (2010).

12 Siegel, *The Mindful Brain*, 46.

Index